Frontiers in Clinical Trials

Edited by Xianli Lv

Published in London, United Kingdom

Frontiers in Clinical Trials
http://dx.doi.org/10.5772/intechopen.104172
Edited by Xianli Lv

Contributors
Teketel Ermias Geltore, Thomas J. FitzGerald, Fran Laurie, Matthew Iandoli, Maryann Bishop-Jodoin, Koren Smith, Kenneth Ulin, Janaki Moni, Maria Giulia Cicchetti, Stephen Kry, Michael Knopp, Ying Xiao, Mark Rosen, Fred Prior, Joel Saltz, Hiroyuki Oura, Go Miyata, Chen Li, Haitao Pan, Ping Huang, Madiha Khan Niazi, Zainab Saeed, Sahar Imran, Farooq Hassan

First published in London, United Kingdom, 2023 by IntechOpen
IntechOpen is the global imprint of INTECHOPEN LIMITED, registered in England and Wales, registration number: 11086078, 5 Princes Gate Court, London, SW7 2QJ, United Kingdom

British Library Cataloguing-in-Publication Data
A catalogue record for this book is available from the British Library

Additional hard and PDF copies can be obtained from orders@intechopen.com

Frontiers in Clinical Trials
Edited by Xianli Lv
p. cm.
Print ISBN 978-1-83768-068-9
Online ISBN 978-1-83768-069-6
eBook (PDF) ISBN 978-1-83768-070-2

For EU product safety concerns:
IN TECH d.o.o., Prolaz Marije Krucifikse Kozulić 3, 51000 Rijeka, Croatia,
info@intechopen.com or visit our website at intechopen.com.

Meet the editor

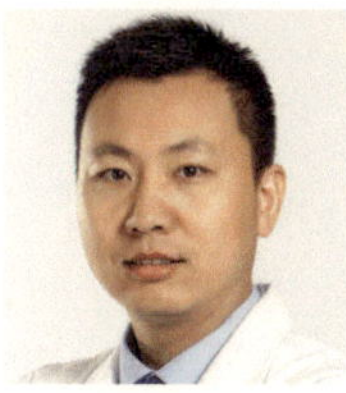

Dr. Xianli Lv, MD, is an associate professor in the Department of Neurosurgery, Beijing Tsinghua Changgung Hospital, School of Clinical Medicine, Tsinghua University, China. His research focuses on neuroendovascular therapy of intracranial aneurysms, cerebral arteriovenous malformation, intracranial dural arteriovenous fistula, spinal vascular malformation, and pediatric cerebrospinal vascular malformation. He has one national invention patent to his credit and has authored 195 peer-reviewed scientific articles and edited 6 books. He is an editorial member of *Interventional Neuroradiology*, *Stroke and Vascular Neurology*, *Journal of Neuroradiology*, *Neuroradiology Journal*, and *World Journal of Radiology*. He is also a deputy editor of *Neuroscience Informatics* and *Frontiers in Neurology*. Dr. Lv is a member of the World Stroke Organization (WSO) and the World Federation of Interventional Therapeutic Neuroradiology (WFITN) and a technical consultant for BALT, Montmorency, France. He was featured on the cover of the *World Journal of Radiology* in April 2022.

Contents

Preface

The knowledge-driven medical research paradigm is encountering bottlenecks. A paradigm refers to a collection of academic elements that are commonly followed by a scientific community. These elements include values, basic theories, laws and regulations, practical norms, technical standards, and exemplary examples. Since the Renaissance, medical research has mainly formed two paradigms: a knowledge-driven research paradigm and a problem-driven research paradigm. The former has always played an important role in the development of medical systems. Under this paradigm, medicine is divided into independent knowledge systems. Medical subdivisions accelerate the creation, accumulation, iteration, and sublimation of knowledge, and promote the systematic construction and improvement of medical knowledge systems. In a relatively closed discipline system, researchers, motivated by their curiosity and thirst for knowledge, freely think about and choose topics for research, emphasize the non-utilitarian and non-social attributes of knowledge, and recognize that the progress of theoretical knowledge has endless application prospects. This innovation model driven by knowledge exploration has promoted the development of modern medicine and the progress of human health care. The well-known milestones of modern medicine, such as the theory of evolution, cell theory, and the principle of life center, are all important academic products under the knowledge-driven research paradigm.

The physiological function and pathological changes of the human body are highly complex. From molecules, cells, tissues, organs, and systems to the human body, these system functions are regulated by multiple factors in a multidimensional manner and depend on the nonlinear interaction between components. It is difficult to reveal and analyze the complex physiological and pathological mechanisms and evolution laws of the human body using traditional research methods dominated by reductionism. In the face of the medical problems of complex diseases such as malignant tumors, cardiovascular and cerebrovascular diseases, and coexistence of multiple diseases brought about by the aging society, the existing research models, such as fragmentation, low dimension, and reductionism, are even more difficult to use to make major breakthroughs.

Obviously, the knowledge-driven scientific research paradigm has formed disciplinary barriers between knowledge systems, resulting in the lack of systematic thinking and methods in scientific research, encountering difficulties in solving complex medical problems, and significantly weakening the contribution to social economy. The further tilt of biomedical research investment has not brought significant improvement in people's well-being.

In addition, another reason the knowledge-driven paradigm is so controversial is that it relies on such indicators as papers, academic qualifications, and academic titles as evaluation criteria. From the statistical data, with the advance of the years, scientific research investment was carried out according to the knowledge-driven model. The value of medical research can be embodied and disseminated through papers, but papers should not be the purpose of medical research. We need papers because they can help more peers share and apply valuable knowledge and technology to benefit patients.

The problem-driven medical research paradigm is gaining acceptance quietly. In this paradigm, "problems" play the leading role in research. Here, "problems" refer to the practical problems that restrict social and economic development. Therefore, academic research under the problem-driven scientific research paradigm has a strong social attribute and utilitarian color. It is not for the sake of improving the knowledge system of a single discipline but is more focused on whether to solve the problems in social and economic development. The goal is to meet practical needs by developing new and practical scientific and technological products, and thus this paradigm is more suitable for interdisciplinary systematic research.

This problem-solving research can generate rich and useful knowledge in theory and technology, stimulate the development of relevant traditional disciplines, and promote the generation of new interdisciplinary and marginal disciplines through "discipline interaction." Compared with knowledge-driven research, the evaluation criteria of problem-driven research are more diversified, and need to be judged from two basic aspects: practicality (usefulness) and scientificity (rationality). It depends not only on published research papers but also on the academic, social, and economic values of scientific research achievements. It also depends on what benefits a medical research achievement really brings to patients and what benefits it creates for the social healthcare service system. "Research without innovation is nonsense, research without products is futile," which fully reflects the core values of the problem-driven research paradigm.

The problem of people's health needs is the main battlefield of current medical research. Scientific research separated from clinical problems is a tree without roots and water without a source. Clinical problem-driven research (CDR) is a way to identify problems through clinical practice and then define the scientific and technical problems therein. Carrying out clinical research or transforming medical or scientific research results in the development of diagnosis and treatment standards and products, practice guidelines, innovative drugs, medical equipment, and more for clinical verification, evaluation, and optimization.

The era of the knowledge economy has higher requirements for "integration of science, technology and economy." Therefore, under the CDR paradigm, we also emphasize the health product-oriented (Bedside to Bench to Clients, B2B2C) research and development model. The ultimate goal of clinical research is not to publish papers, but to produce health technology products with practical value, providing inexhaustible momentum for the sustainable development of the health industry, so as to form clinical research. The positive interaction between medical practice and industrial development is a closed loop.

Therefore, medical science and technology innovation will gradually shift from a knowledge-driven research paradigm to a clinical-driven research paradigm. At present, a new round of scientific and technological revolution and industrial transformation is reshaping the global innovation landscape and economic structure. Scientific and technological innovation is characterized by intersection, integration, penetration, and radiation. Disruptive technological innovation is constantly emerging. Scientific big data is becoming a new scientific research model following experimental science, theoretical analysis, and computer simulation. System medicine with data intelligence as the core technology in the medical field will strongly promote the steady development of CDR characterized by disciplinary integration and systematic research.

Academic physicians are leaders in clinical-driven research. Clinicians are on the front line of clinical practice and are the primary discoverers of clinical problems. An outstanding academic clinician should always take scientific and technological innovation as their mission and responsibility for career development, and should not be satisfied with treating patients only with existing knowledge. We should pursue knowledge creation and technology innovation and play a leading and integrated role in clinical research. Through the research strategy of "finding problems, initiating research, establishing projects by consensus, communication and cooperation, finding good strategies, and applying evaluation," we should solve the problems and pain points in practical health care and continue to improve the level of medical services and quality of care for patients.

As an endovascular neurosurgeon, I also have some ideas about the growth and development of academic doctors. Surgical clinical work is faced with the challenge of complex and difficult diseases that cannot be solved by traditional clinical thinking and surgical methods. Behind the clinical challenges are the scientific and technical issues in surgical practice. In terms of scientific issues, it is necessary to seek systematic intervention rules for multi-objective optimization, and in terms of technical issues, it is necessary to explore deterministic intervention technologies to achieve multi-objective optimization. Through clinical research, we established the maximum intersection theory, namely, the three elements balance rule, under the collaborative constraint of seeking lesion clearance, nerve protection, and nerve damage control. At the same time, we have carried out innovation and practice of deterministic neuro-interventional technology, using visualization, quantification, and controllability technology to overcome factors that are difficult to determine, predict, and control in traditional empirical neuro-interventional clinical practice. We achieved a balance of three elements in clinical practice with accurate decision-making and application of appropriate intervention methods to obtain safe, efficient, and minimally invasive multi-objective optimization. The ultimate goal is to maximize the health benefits of patients.

Based on the exploration and practice of continuously improving the effect of endovascular therapy for complex cerebral and spinal vascular diseases, I put forward the concept of "precision endovascular neurosurgery," built a precision endovascular neurosurgery paradigm, solved a series of difficult endovascular therapy problems for complex cerebral and spinal vascular diseases, and promoted the level of endovascular neurosurgery.

Lao Tzu of *Tao Te Ching* says, "A tree that is hugged is born at the end of a centimeter; a platform of nine layers begins with a pile of earth; a journey of a thousand miles begins with a single step." It is the responsibility and mission of clinicians to lead clinical-driven research. The process from clinical practice to theoretical and technological innovation is also an important transition process for clinicians from "craftsman" to "home." Clinical-driven research must be supported by the innovative system of academic hospitals. At present, under the clinical problem-driven research paradigm, medical research and medical services are often "two skins." There are still many problems between them, such as differences in professional direction, lack of cooperation channels, difficulties in transformation and application, and contradictions in achievement sharing. There is an urgent need to reconstruct the organizational model and ecosystem of medical science and technology innovation and the links between basic research, clinical research, transformation research, and industrialization.

We would like to thank all the authors for their contributions. We would also like to acknowledge the encouragement, motivation, and assistance from the Beijing Municipal Administration of Hospitals Incubating Program (PX2020039), China, and Tsinghua Precision Medicine Foundation (20219990008), Tsinghua University, Beijing, China.

Xianli Lv
Neurosurgery Department,
Beijing Tsinghua Changgung Hospital,
School of Clinical Medicine,
Tsinghua University,
Beijing, China

Section 1

Design of Clinical Trial

Chapter 1

Introduction to Bayesian Group Sequential Design

Chen Li, Ping Huang and Haitao Pan

Abstract

In classical group sequential designs, a clinical trial is considered as a success if the experimental treatment is statistically significantly better than placebo. The criteria for stopping or continuing the trial are chosen to control the false-positive rate (type I error). Bayesian group sequential design has an advantage of allowing inclusion of prior information in the analysis. The decision criteria can be based on the posterior or predictive distribution of the treatment effect to stop for success or futility, or to continue for each interim analysis and the final analysis. This chapter introduces Bayesian group sequential designs with examples in a confirmatory setting, including how to calibrate the tuning parameters to set up decision criteria for the interim and final analyses, how to derive the sample size, and how to evaluate the operating characteristics via simulations.

Keywords: Bayesian, group sequential design, prior, effective sample size, decision-making

1. Introduction

In confirmatory trials, randomized controlled trials (RCTs) are the gold standard for treatment evaluation, which directly compare the investigational drug with the standard treatment or a placebo (if there is no standard of care). The essential component for a trial design is to find the sample size that is necessary to detect a clinically important treatment difference with sufficient power and controlled type I error rate. Once all observations have been collected, final analyses will be conducted. However, due to lack of information on both the magnitude and the sampling variability of the new treatment effect at the design stage, realized sample size may be different from what the design gives use. To that end, the fixed designs can be inefficient since they cannot accommodate this discrepancy.

There has been an increasing interest in group sequential designs that can adapt to the information collected during the process of the trial. In contrast to fixed designs, group sequential methods are flexible and adaptive to regularly examine the efficacy over administratively convenient time intervals [1]. During the process of a trial, strong evidence in favor of the benefit of the novel treatment may emerge early. If so, the extra study participants required to provide this protection against a false-negative result may not be necessary. Stopping the trial before the maximum planned sample size can save

IntechOpen

resources and accelerate the trial process. Of course, this advantage must be balanced against the potential for the overestimation of the treatment effect and other limitations of smaller trials (e.g. limited safety data and less information about treatment effects in subgroups). Conversely, if strong evidence accumulating against the benefit of the new treatment, it would be unethical for patients continuing to be exposed to the futility therapy. Interim analysis is a useful tool to stop trials early for futility. In classical frequentist group sequential designs, the criteria for stopping or continuing the trial are chosen to control the type I error and p-values are used to make decisions.

Rather than making inference by using p-values, criteria for success and futility stopping, Go/No-go decisions in Bayesian design are based on the posterior probability (PoP) or posterior predictive probability (PreP) at the interim and final analyses [2, 3]. Based on these statistical tools, use of the cumulating data through interim analyses allows the trial design adapted to improve design efficiency. For example, ineffective treatment arms could be dropped; further treatment arms could be introduced; the trial could be stopped early (due to futility/efficacy); or randomization to treatment could be altered to favor the more effective treatment. Such adaptations are attractive to both researchers and patients, by making more efficient use of patient resource and potentially treating patients more effectively. In general, adaptive clinical trial designs are easier to implement within the Bayesian framework. Frequentist designs may not always work. While, Bayesian methods have particular advantage in rare disease scenarios where traditional methods can be difficult, if not impossible, to achieve due to limited sample size. To that end, the Bayesian approach is that they allow inclusion of external information, which can be historical, nonconcurrent information. By applying dynamic borrowing methods or matching approaches to create a synthetical control arm or augment a control arm, sample size may be saved.

In this chapter, we provide an introduction of Bayesian group sequential trials and discuss some commonly used design features with an example.

2. The decision rule in classical frequentist framework

Classical group sequential trials rely on null hypothesis testing involving calculation of test statistics, along with p-values and confidence intervals. The critical statistical issue with early stopping, particularly for success, is accounting for multiple "looks" and repeatedly testing the null hypothesis over time. However, the more frequently the data analyzed, the greater the chance of observing one of these fluctuations. Therefore, the decision criteria for early stopping or continuing the trial are chosen to control the overall type I error rate (e.g. 0.05) [4, 5]. For example, the null ($H_0 : \delta \leq 0$) and alternative ($H_0 : \delta > 0$) hypotheses are formulated for the true treatment difference δ (large values of δ correspond to a positive effect) in a two-arm trials, and the type I error (α) is set to a specified value. The null hypothesis will be rejected if the observed one-sided p-value is less than . The interim analysis can be performed on a specific calendar date within the planning period of times, which is called calendar time. It can also be performed at the information time, which is a predefined proportion of maximum subjects or events/outcomes already observed, especially in time-to-event trials. To account for multiple testing on several interim analyses, interim hypothesis testing always based on α-spending functions, such as Pocock method and O'Brien-Fleming method [6]. The stopping rules require a very small p-value smaller than the false-positive rate boundaries in the interims. The more conservative the early stopping criteria, the more assurance there is that an early stop for success is not a false-positive result.

3. The decision rule in Bayesian perspectives

Unlike frequentist approaches where parameters of interest are considered deterministic, the parameters in the Bayesian paradigm are treated as random, while the data collected in the trial have been observed and thus considered fixed. The prior distributions that we assign to the unknown interest parameters (e.g. treatment effect) can be viewed as our uncertainty initial belief about them. Once data of the current trial collected, new information becomes available and is summarized by another distribution—the likelihood. Using Bayes' theorem, the prior can be combined with the likelihood and updated to become a posterior distribution. Accordingly, various posterior probabilities and inferences can be drawn. Thus, the decision can be made by the posterior probabilities which summarize all information available at that point in time. We can find the empirical frequentist error rates for a Bayesian testing procedure by fixing certain parameter boundaries at prespecified values. Bayesian approach provides an alternative statistical framework and uses probability distributions to represent uncertainty of the parameter estimation. By carefully calibrating design parameters, not only do the methods enhance flexibility of trial conduct and monitoring, but they can also maintain the frequentist type I and type II error rates at the nominal levels.

From a Bayesian perspective, the decision-making is based on the PoP for the treatment effect given the trial data. If the PoP for the interest parameter δ beyond the effect threshold s is sufficiently high, i.e. above a prespecified boundary θ_s, denoted by $Pr(\delta > s|D) \geq \theta_s$, the trial could allow for early stopping for efficacy. By the same token, early stopping for futility may be permitted if the PoP is below the futility boundary θ_f, expressed as $Pr(\delta > s|D) \leq \theta_f$. If the probability falls between these two values θ_s and θ_f, then the trial may continue recruiting. Since the Bayesian methods are not required for multiple looks corrections, the decision can be made at any time with the updating PoP. Also, the stopping rules in each interim can be constructed independently and multiple criteria can be required based on several treatment effect thresholds. For example, the success criteria of a trial can be quantified as:

$$Pr(\delta > s_1|D) \geq \theta_{s1} \; and \; Pr(\delta > s_2|D) \geq \theta_{s2}. \tag{1}$$

where s_1 and s_2 are specified effect thresholds, and θ_{s1} and θ_{s2} are specified or tuned probability boundaries. The multiple quantitative criteria based on the PoP may greatly help to achieve a clinically meaningful decision-making. This is appealing to clinicians and statisticians who will often want to know how a given design will conclude in favor of some particular treatment effects.

Although the type I error and power are frequentist concepts, the Bayesian approach can calculate something analogous to these quantities for any prespecified decision rules. It can also consider multiple "looks" as the frequentist approach to control the type I error. The multiple corrections, such as based on α-spending functions, may be conducted as the Bayesian early stopping boundaries on the interim analysis to maintain the total false-positive rate. The PoP can also be considered as the power for a specific treatment effect when the target treatment effect is assumed to be the true value. It assists with decision-making to demonstrate that the Bayesian design has good frequentist operating characteristics.

4. Decision boundaries

The decision boundaries for the PoP can be specified based on a clinically meaningful treatment effect threshold by the investigator. For example, one can stop for efficacy if the PoP of having a hazard ratio (HR) <1 above 90%, i.e. $Pr(HR < 1|D) > 0.9$, and one can stop for futility if $Pr(HR < 1|D) < 0.2$. In practice, however, Bayesian designs usually rely on simulations to determine the decision boundaries and parameter calibration. This is achieved by determining how frequently the Bayesian design incorrectly declares a treatment to be effective or superior when it is assumed that there is truly no difference. It has often been used to tune stopping boundaries to ensure acceptable type I error, e.g. 2.5% one-sided type I error or 5% two-sided type I error. The power for a specific treatment effect can be calculated as the proportion of simulations that declare the trial to be "successful" when the target treatment effect is assumed to be the true value. This approach has been recommended by the FDA [4] and has been used in practice for Bayesian adaptive designs [7, 8]. These simulations should be performed in the planning stage of a Bayesian group sequential trail. In the analysis stage, no further adjustments are required to account for the previous interim analyses that have been performed.

We use a simulations study to introduce how to obtain the decision boundaries. Consider a two-arm RCT with two interim analyses, and a final analysis is planned with time-to-event outcomes, such as progression-free survival (PFS) times. Let T denote the underlying failure time, which may be right-censored, and let C denote the censoring time. We denote the observed time as $X = \min(T, C)$ with a censoring indicator $\Delta = I(T \leq C)$, i.e. if $\Delta = 1$ then $X = T$, which is the failure time, and if $\Delta = 0$, then $X = C$, which is the censoring time. We assume the survival times for both the treatment and placebo arms followed exponential distributions with means of μ_T and μ_C, respectively. The null hypothesis is equivalence of the two treatments in terms of the efficacy, and the alternative hypothesis is the treatment better than the control. Under the exponential survival model, the mean survival time is the reciprocal of the hazard, that is, the hazard ratio (HR) = μ_C/μ_T and a lower value means better treatment. It could be claimed success if HR between two groups given the observed data D satisfies

$$Pr\left(\log\left(\frac{\mu_C}{\mu_T}\right) < \delta|D\right) > \theta_T \tag{2}$$

where δ is an effect threshold for a clinically meaningful treatment difference, and θ_T is a probability boundary for decision-making.

In the Bayesian framework, we specify a prior distribution for the mean survival time μ following an inverse-gamma (IG) prior distribution for μ:

$$\mu \sim IG(\alpha, \beta) = \frac{\beta^{\alpha}}{\Gamma(\alpha)}\mu^{-\alpha-1}\exp(-\beta/\mu) \tag{3}$$

where $\alpha > 0$ and $\beta > 0$. Since the IG distribution is conjugate with the exponential likelihood function, the posterior distribution of μ also follows an IG distribution:

$$p(\mu|D) \propto \mu^{-\sum_{i=1}^{n}\Delta_i - \alpha - 1}\exp\left(-\frac{\sum_{i=1}^{n}x_i + \beta}{\mu}\right) \tag{4}$$

That is, $\mu|D\propto IG\left(\sum_{i=1}^{n}\Delta_i + \alpha,\ \sum_{i=1}^{n}x_i + \beta\right)$. Thus, we can compute the PoP of the treatment better than the control as shown in Eq.(1). If $PoP > \theta_T$, we claim the treatment superior to the control. We should also specify the lower and upper probability boundaries θ_L and θ_U for decision-making in interim analysis. The decision rules in the interim analysis are given as follows:

1. *Success stopping* If $Pr\left(\log\left(\frac{\mu_C}{\mu_T}\right) < \delta|D\right) > \theta_U$, we stop the trial to claim a superior treatment.

2. *Futility stopping* If $Pr\left(\log\left(\frac{\mu_C}{\mu_T}\right) < \delta|D\right) < \theta_L$, we stop the trial to claim a futility treatment.

Then, the design parameters (θ_T,θ_U,θ_L) can be calibrated via simulation to achieve desirable trial operating characteristics.

5. Parameter calibration and setup

The parameters calibration needs two stages.

In stage 1, we focus on choosing an appropriate probability boundary θ_T for the specific treatment effect δ. We simulate the data under a "null" scenario of HR = 1 to calibrate the parameter that can control the false-positive rate. In this step, we firstly set $\theta_L = 1$ and $\theta_U = 0$ such that the trial will not be terminate early. Considering null hypothesis $H_0 : \mu_T = \mu_C$ and the alternative hypothesis $H_1 : \mu_T = \mu_C \times e^{\delta}$, an initial sample size can be obtained by the frequentist method. Let the prior distribution of μ for each arms be non-informative prior such as IG (0.01,0.01) and simulate the data under the null hypothesis. We simulate millions of trials and count the number of trials that were declared to be successful in which the decision rule was shown in Eq.1. The proportion of trials that were successful when assuming a HR = 1 provides the simulated type I error rate. Then we vary the value of θ_T (e.g. from 0.6 to 0.95) and calculate the PoP in Eq.1 $Pr(\log HR < \delta|D) > \theta_T$. If the final PoP is higher than the given type I error, it means that the probability boundary is too loose to control the false-positive rate, and we should increase θ_T and use more stringent stopping boundaries. On the contrary, if PoP is lower than the given type I error, θ_T can be decreased to loosen the efficacy stopping boundaries. Until PoP is close to the type I error, the corresponding θ_T can be chosen as the final efficacy success boundary.

In the second stage, we fixed the chosen θ_T in stage 1 and varied the value of θ_U and θ_L, such as $\theta_U = 0.90, \ldots 0.99$ and $\theta_L = 0.01, \ldots 0.10$, to calibrate early stopping boundaries in the interim analysis. Similar to the calibration procedures in stage 1, we select the appropriate combination of θ_U and θ_L to control the given type I error with simulations presented above.

6. Sample size estimation

In this step, based on the above calibrated parameters (θ_T,θ_U,θ_L), we simulate the data under the alternative hypothesis using the initial sample size estimated by the frequentist method. The proportion of the simulation trials declared to be successful based on the given decision criteria can be interpreted as the conditional power. If it is lower than the given power, it means the current sample sizes cannot provide adequate power, and we should increase sample size and vice versa. Until the PoP reaches to the given power, the corresponding sample sizes can be finally determined.

7. Prior distribution and ESS

Although noninformative prior has been widely applied in the design stage, the prior can also be constructed using domain knowledge based on expert clinical opinion or information from previous studies. Borrowing data on the control arm may result in a more efficiently design and more favorable operating characteristics by way of a smaller trial overall or patients on the control arm. Although the idea of using historical data is not new, proper application is critical. Challenges exist in quantifying the level of relevance of historical data. When incorporating prior information, it is significant to choose prior beliefs into trials. For example, we can use skeptical or enthusiastic priors to decide partial or fully borrowing of the external information. In practice, to utilize historical data as enthusiastic prior data for the current trials, it must be assumed that the historical data are fully relevant to this trial patient population. If unsure of the relevance of prior information, a probability of relevance can be incorporated as part of the prior distribution, such as

$$\text{prior} = (1 - \alpha) * f(D) + \alpha * g(D) \tag{5}$$

where f(D) is skeptical prior distribution (the external information or historical data are completely different from current data), g(D) is the enthusiastic prior distribution (historical data reflects current data) and relevance factor, and α is the applicability probability of current data [9]. A number between 0 and 1 for the relevance factor α corresponds to the amount of information borrowed from the historical data, that is, the interpretation of applicability of the historical data. Some other common methods for discounting are weighted average of the means for the randomized and historical controls to control bias, such as the power prior approach [10], the commensurate prior approach [11], meta-analytic predictive (MAP) approaches [12], and so on. Modeling and simulation are useful tools to explore and set expectations on the relevance of the historical data. Even if prior information seems very relevant, sufficient skepticism about potential efficacy exists; therefore, requiring that prior information should be discounted.

Quantification of the amount of information induced by the prior is important to avoid domination of the prior information on posterior inference. The effective sample size (ESS) reflects the amount of borrowing by incorporating prior information, which equates prior information to a certain number of observations. Since the historical information may not be commensurate with the information collected during the current trial, there may be a prior-data conflict observed. The ESS can quantify the strength of prior information and its contributions to the inference.

Prior effective sample sizes are well understood for conjugate of one-parameter exponential families. It can be motivated in the updating rule from prior to posterior parameters. For example, for Poisson data with a $Gamma(a, b)$ prior, the second parameter of the posterior Gamma distribution is $b + n$, implying b as the prior ESS. In another way, the posterior mean is a weighted average of the prior mean and the standard parameter estimate, with weights proportional to the prior ESS and the sample size n. For Poisson data, the prior mean and parameter estimate are a/b and $\sum Y_j/n$, and the posterior mean $(a + \sum Y_j)/(b + n)$ is the weighted average of the two, with weights proportional to b and n. The ESS under conjugacy can be concluded with different distribution as follow:

Distribution	Prior	ESS
Normal	$Normal(\mu, s^2/n_0)$	n_0
Binary	$Beta(a, b)$	$a + b$
Poisson	$Gamma(a, b)$	b

Another more involved information-based ESS has been suggested in the seminal paper by Morita [13], which has been denoted as Morita method for short. In addition to the Fisher information, it uses the information of the prior distribution $p(\theta)$:

$$\mathrm{i(p(\theta))} = -\frac{\mathrm{d^2 logp(\theta)}}{\mathrm{d\theta^2}} \tag{6}$$

and the information of and ϵ-information (large variance) prior $p_0(\theta)$ with the same mean $(\overline{\theta})$ as$p(\theta)$:

$$\mathrm{i(p_0(\theta))} = -\frac{\mathrm{d^2 \log p_0(\theta)}}{\mathrm{d\theta^2}} \tag{7}$$

The ESS can be defined as an interger m that minimizes the distance (evaluated at the prior mean $\overline{\theta}$) between the expected posterior information for a sample of size m based on the same mean large variance prior $p_0(\theta)$ and the information of the actual prior:

$$|\mathrm{i(p_0(\overline{\theta})) + E_{Y_m}\{i_F(Y_m; \overline{\theta})\} - i(p_0(\theta))}| \tag{8}$$

where the expectation of Y_m is taken over the prior-predictive distribution under $p(\theta)$. This approach is noteworthy because it appears to be the first formal, metric-based approach to ESS that complies with the standard one-parameter exponential family ESS.

There is also another information-based ESS, which is described as expected local-information-ratio (ELIR) method [14]. It also uses the prior and Fisher information, but instead of locally evaluating the respective information ratio at the mean (or mode), and it is defined as the mean of the prior information to Fisher information ratio $r(\theta)$:

$$\mathrm{ESS_{ELIS} = E_\theta\{r(\theta)\} = E_\theta\left\{\frac{i(p(\theta))}{i_F(\theta)}\right\}} \tag{9}$$

ESS_{ELIS} gives the well-known effective sample sizes for some standard one parameter exponential families. For the natural parameter η, it is the standard ESS without any boundary restriction on the parameters. The information ratio $i(\eta) = i(p(\eta))/i_F(\eta)$ does not depend on the parameter. For the natural parameter, the sampling and prior distribution can be written as:

$$f(y|\theta) = \exp\{y\eta - M(\eta)\}, p|(\eta) = \exp\{n_0 m_0 \eta - n_0 M(\eta)\} \tag{10}$$

Since $i_F(\theta) = d^2M(\eta)/d\eta^2$, it follows that $ESS_{ELIS} = n_0$. Take Poisson data for example, with a Gamma prior for the mean μ, $\eta = \log(\mu)$, $M(\eta) = exp(\eta)$ and $n_0 = b$. Therefore, the *ELIS* method seems to be simple and superior to current versions.

8. Example

In the following, we use the above example to illustrate the design of Bayesian group sequential trial. It will be used in a randomized, double-blinded, placebo-controlled study on the efficacy of new treatment to improve the survival in advanced triple-negative breast cancer patients. The primary time-to-event end point is PFS within 30 months. It is allowed for 90% power to detect an improvement in median PFS from 6 months in the control arm to 10 months in the new treatment arm, that is, the target HR = 0.6 with 2.5% level of significance (one-sided). Accrual is projected to occur over 15 months, and the final PFS analysis is expected 30 months after the first patient enrolls. Assuming normal distribution for logHRs, it could be claimed success if the posterior distribution of logHR satisfies $Pr(\log HR < \delta \mid D) > \theta_T$ given the observed data D, and no futility criterion is required at the end of the trial. Considering two interim analyses at approximately 50% and 80% of information fraction, the success and futility early stopping criteria are $Pr(\log HR < \delta \mid D) > \theta_U$ and $Pr(\log HR < \delta|D) < \theta_L$, respectively. Now we need to calibrate the design parameters $(\theta_T, \theta_U, \theta_L)$ for the decision-making.

Firstly, we calculate an initial sample size by classical frequentist method for the simulation. With an average 5% dropout rate per year, there will be approximately 100 patients required in each arm and totally 164 events occurred. Then, we simulate the data under null hypothesis (HR = 1) and did not allow early stopping in the interim analyses. Assuming a non-informative prior distribution of mean survival μ for each arm, e.g., IG (0.01,0.01), we took 5000 posterior samples of μ for the PoP calculation. Varying θ_T from 0.6 to 0.99, we performed simulations to calibrate the cutoff probability values to satisfy 2.5% type I error. For each configuration, we carried out 5000 simulated trials to summarize the operating characteristics. The resulting type I error are presented in **Table 1**. With the decreasing of the target logHR, the success probability boundary also decreased to yield 2.5% for the type I

δ	θ_T	Success probability	Sample size	Total time
log(0.8)	0.7	0.0247	218	23.1796
log(0.7)	0.6	0.0083	208	22.0439
log(0.7)	0.5	0.0157	208	22.0022
log(0.7)	0.46	0.0248	208	22.1248
log(0.7)	0.45	0.0210	209	22.2274
log(0.7)	0.43	0.0200	209	22.1462
log(0.6)	0.25	0.0118	190	20.1316
log(0.6)	0.2	0.0123	189	20.0138
log(0.6)	0.18	0.0227	188	19.8901

Table 1.
Stage 1 parameter calibration with no early stopping by varying the design parameter θ_T at different values of δ under null hypothesis with HR = 1.

δ	θ_T	θ_L	θ_U	Success probability	Sample size	Total time
log(0.6)	0.18	0.01	0.91	0.0245	219	17.0610
		0.01	0.93	0.0228	218	16.8673
log(0.7)	0.46	0.01	0.89	0.0236	200	19.8338
		0.01	0.91	0.0328	214	20.2497

Table 2.
Stage 2 parameter calibration with the tuned θ_T by varying the design parameter θ_L and θ_U under null hypothesis.

error. For example, when δ is expected to be $\log(0.7)$, we should select the cutoff value of $\theta_T = 0.46$. When the target HR decreased to 0.6, the boundary decreased sharply to 0.18 to maintain the type I error. So the investigator can choose a clinical meaningful treatment as the target value δ, and multiple criteria can be also required based on several probabilities.

In the second stage of parameter calibration, given a specific δ and the tuned θ_T, we varied the value of θ_U and θ_L: $\theta_U = 0.90, \ldots 0.99$ and $\theta_L = 0.01, \ldots 0.10$. To control the type I error, we finally selected $\theta_U = 0.89$ and $\theta_L = 0.01$ to calibrate early stopping in the interim analysis under the null to detect the effect size of log (HR = 0.7). Similarly, if we want to detect log(HR = 0.6), we should select $\theta_U = 0.91$ and $\theta_L = 0.01$ under the null to control the type I error rate (**Table 2**).

Then, we obtained the tuned parameters (θ_T,θ_U,θ_L) for a specific effect size of . To maintain 90% power, we simulate data from the H_1, e.g. logHR= $\delta = 0.6$, and the expected number of events was found to be 172.

9. Conclusion

In this chapter, we introduce the Bayesian group sequential framework with an example with details for planning and executing interim analyses. The concepts of PoP and predictive probability are intuitive and efficient tools for making decisions about continuation or early stopping and can be used at interim analyses even if the final planned analysis is to be performed in the classical frequentist hypothesis testing framework. Simulations can help assess the performance of different decision rules and assist in the determination of the sample size and are needed to tune desirable design's parameters. Bayesian approaches are often simpler to interpret than frequentist methods and allow teams to consider the evidence in support of different effects. Using these methods in clinical drug development can result in efficient studies that make the best use of resources while ensuring good chances of success. Li's work was partially supported by National Natural Science Foundation of China Grant 82273728.

Author details

Chen Li[1*†], Ping Huang[2†] and Haitao Pan[3]

1 Department of Health Statistics, School of Preventive Medicine, Fourth Military Medical University, Xi'an, Shaanxi, P. R. China

2 State Key Laboratory of Military Stomotology, National Clinical Research Center for Oral Diseases, Shaanxi Clinical Research Center for Oral Diseases, Department of Clinical Laboratory of Stomatology, Fourth Military Medical University, Xi'an, Shaanxi, China

3 Department of Biostatistics, St. Jude Children's Research Hospital, Memphis, TN, USA

*Address all correspondence to: lc.biosta@qq.com

† These authors contributed equally.

References

[1] Lai TL, Lavori PW, Tsang KW. Adaptive design of confirmatory trials: Advances and challenges. Contemporary Clinical Trials. 2015;**45**(Pt A):93-102

[2] Gsponer T, Gerber F, Bornkamp B, Ohlssen D, Vandemeulebroecke M, Schmidli H. A practical guide to Bayesian group sequential designs. Pharmaceutical Statistics. 2014;**13**(1):71-80

[3] Yin G, Lam CK, Shi H. Bayesian randomized clinical trials: From fixed to adaptive design. Contemporary Clinical Trials. 2017;**59**:77-86

[4] FDA. Adaptive Design Clinical Trials for Drugs and Biologics Guidance for Industry. FDA; 2019. Available from: https://www.fda.gov/regulatory-information/search-fda-guidance-documents/adaptive-design-clinical-trials-drugs-and-biologics-guidance-industry

[5] Vandemeulebroecke M. Group sequential and adaptive designs - a review of basic concepts and points of discussion. Biometrical Journal Biometrische Zeitschrift. 2008;**50**(4):541-557

[6] Kittelson JM, Emerson SS. A unifying family of group sequential test designs. Biometrics. 1999;**55**(3):874-882

[7] Connor JT, Elm JJ, Broglio KR. Bayesian adaptive trials offer advantages in comparative effectiveness trials: An example in status epilepticus. Journal of Clinical Epidemiology. 2013;**66**(8 Suppl):S130-S137

[8] Nogueira RG, Jadhav AP, Haussen DC, Bonafe A, Budzik RF, Bhuva P, et al. Thrombectomy 6 to 24 hours after stroke with a mismatch between deficit and infarct. The New England Journal of Medicine. 2018;**378**(1):11-21

[9] Greenhouse JB, Wasserman L. Robust Bayesian methods for monitoring clinical trials. Statistics in Medicine. 1995;**14**(12):1379-1391

[10] Ibrahim JG, Chen MH, Gwon Y, Chen F. The power prior: Theory and applications. Statistics in Medicine. 2015;**34**(28):3724-3749

[11] Hobbs BP, Carlin BP, Mandrekar SJ, Sargent DJ. Hierarchical commensurate and power prior models for adaptive incorporation of historical information in clinical trials. Biometrics. 2011;**67**(3):1047-1056

[12] Schmidli H, Gsteiger S, Roychoudhury S, O'Hagan A, Spiegelhalter D, Neuenschwander B. Robust meta-analytic-predictive priors in clinical trials with historical control information. Biometrics. 2014;**70**(4):1023-1032

[13] Morita S, Thall PF, Müller P. Determining the effective sample size of a parametric prior. Biometrics. 2008;**64**(2):595-602

[14] Neuenschwander B, Weber S, Schmidli H, O'Hagan A. Predictively consistent prior effective sample sizes. Biometrics. 2020;**76**(2):578-587

Section 2

Clinical Trials

Chapter 2

Benefits of Organizational Anger Management Program to Prevent Disruptive Behaviors: A Japanese Hospital Case Study

Hiroyuki Oura and Go Miyata

Abstract

Intervention to inhibit disruptive behavior (DB) in healthcare institutions remains an unmet need. This study intended to examine the feasibility of an organizational anger management (AM) program aimed at inhibiting DB triggered by anger. AM dissemination and awareness-building activities for all staff members (1366 individuals) were implemented from July 2020, including regularly held group AM introductory trainings, establishment of "I Will Not Get Angry Today" days (once per month), posting of AM promotion posters in all departments (changed monthly), disseminating AM-related knowledge through the in-hospital groupware application (twice per week), and introduction of AM training methods using the in-hospital periodical magazine. The number of responses to the awareness survey questionnaire 1 year after AM program was 730 (response rate: 54.2%). The results showed that the percentage of positive responses indicating that DB "Decreased" or "Somewhat Decreased" after AM program intervention was 35.8% overall. The percentages for nurses (n = 385) and non-nurses (n = 345) groups were 29.8% and 42.4%, respectively, showing a significantly lower value for nurses ($p < 0.001$). An organizational AM program aimed at inhibiting DB could be implemented at our facility. However, it was difficult to properly evaluate the efficacy due to the nature of the study.

Keywords: disruptive behavior, anger management, patient safety, psychological safety, medical institution

1. Introduction

Problematic behaviors such as swearing, ranting, and personal attacks by healthcare professionals are referred to as disruptive behavior (DB) [1, 2]. It is well known that DB causes mental stress to the victimized staff members, inducing errors due to decreased motivation and alertness. Furthermore, DB leads to medical accidents because of communication failures and labor shortages as a result of high turnover of nursing staff and deterioration of psychological safety [3–5]. The large-scale study by Rosenstein and Daniel [4] on VHA West Coast hospitals revealed that of all the physicians and nurses who participated in the survey, 97% experienced DB at work. A total of 71% of them felt that DB could lead to a medical accident, and 27% recognized that DB could lead to the death of a patient. A survey of hospital managers by the American College of Physician Executives [6] found that 71% of the hospital managers were aware that DB occurred on a monthly basis in each hospital, and more than 11% were aware that it occurred daily. In addition, 99% of them stated that DB had a negative effect on medical care, and 21% felt that it caused a disadvantage to the patients.

Thus, DB has long been understood as a serious threat to patient safety and hospital management. In particular, various measures have been taken against disruptive physician behavior [7–9], but at present, sufficient efficacy has not been realized. Furthermore, it is well known that DB can occur not only with physicians but also with many other medical professionals such as nurses and pharmacists [10–12]. However, almost no measures for prevention have been taken in this regard [13]. To date, little research has been conducted on DB intervention, and DB management in medical institutions remains an unmet need.

In the medical field, where lives are at stake, staff members are exposed to various forms of intense stress each day, which can increase the likelihood of a reaction of anger, and is one of the factors that causes DB to occur frequently [10, 12–14]. In August 2019, we conducted on all staff members (1376 persons) of our hospital, an advanced acute care hospital, a survey on the actual condition of in-hospital DB (DB cases that occurred in the past 6 months; number of responses: 346; response rate: 25.1%). The results revealed that of the 365 reported cases of DB, DB that was thought to be triggered by anger accounted for 65% of all DB cases (total of 236 cases), including 123 cases of "Being screamed at and emotionally criticized." Anger was the largest factor for the occurrence of DB. These results suggested that an organizational AM program may be effective in inhibiting DB.

To the authors' knowledge, there have been no reports on organizational AM programs aimed at inhibiting DB in medical institutions. Hence, the present study intended to examine the feasibility of an organizational AM program to inhibit DB.

2. Materials and methods

After the in-hospital implementation project team for the AM program was launched in May 2020, the lead author, who acted as the team leader, obtained the Certified Anger Management Specialist-I qualification from the National Anger Management Association. From July of the same year, AM dissemination and awareness-building activities were initiated for all staff members, including part-time staff (1366 people). The categorization of staff members by occupation was as follows: 688 nurses (50.4%), 205 physicians (15.0%), 35 pharmacists (2.6%), 148 technicians (10.8%), 118 clerical staff (8.6%), and 172 other occupations (12.6%).

AM dissemination and awareness-building methods consisted of the following initiatives. First, group AM introductory training for all staff members was conducted regularly. This introductory training was imparted in accordance with the program for beginner-level AM training participants established by the Japan Chapter of the National Anger Management Association. Next, an "I Will Not Get Angry Today" declaration day was established (the first Monday of each month), and by posting "Declaration Day" awareness-raising posters in all departments of the hospital at all times, the first Monday of each month was made an opportunity to be aware of one's feelings of anger. An announcement was broadcast twice (once in the morning and once in the afternoon) in the entire facility on the "Declaration Day." Additionally, AM promotion posters were posted in all departments, with the training method's theme changed each month. The posters were posted with particular emphasis on places where DB frequently occurs, such as the emergency room, operating room, and catheter room. Also, AM-related knowledge was disseminated by the in-hospital groupware application twice weekly, which could be viewed by the staff members. Lastly, the AM training methods were introduced in the periodic in-hospital public relations magazine. Participation in AM programs, such as the introductory training, was not obligatory, and it was left to the discretion of each staff member.

In July 2021 (the 13th month after the start of the AM program), an awareness survey questionnaire was administered to all employees (1348 individuals) to evaluate the efficacy of the organizational AM program with regard to inhibition of DB (**Table 1**). The questionnaire was administered in an anonymous manner, and personal information was strictly managed so that the respondents could not be identified. The responses to the awareness survey questionnaire were aggregated based on the occupation, divided into two groups (nurses and non-nurses), and the response selection ratios for each question were compared. Regarding the method of intergroup comparative analysis of the response selection ratio, a z-test was used to analyze the difference in the unpaired population ratios. A two-tailed test was used for statistical hypothesis testing, and the significance level was set to a risk rate of <5%. IBM SPSS 25.0 J for Windows was used for statistical processing. In the intergroup comparison analysis, Questions 1 and 2 were analyzed using the response

Administered to all staff members in July 2021 (13th month after the program start)	
	Details of questions:
Question 1.	Do you know about anger management? 1. I know about it 2. I have heard about it, but do not know much 3. I do not know about it
Question 2.	Do you practice anger management? 1. I practice it on a regular basis 2. I have practiced it but mostly do not practice it 3. I have never practiced it
Question 3.	Do you think that disruptive behavior in your department has decreased since the start of the organizational anger management program? 1. Decreased 2. Somewhat decreased 3. Not sure 4. Somewhat increased 5. Increased
Question 4.	Do you think that an organizational anger management program can help control disruptive behavior? 1. Effective 2. Somewhat effective 3. Not sure 4. Ineffective
Question 5.	Would you like to recommend anger management training to your family members and acquaintances? 1. Would recommend 2. Would somewhat recommend 3. Not sure 4. Would not recommend
Question 6.	What are your thoughts on the organizational anger management program (free response)?

Table 1.
Awareness survey on the inhibitive effects of an organizational anger management program on disruptive behavior.

selection ratios of the Top Box and Bottom Box. Q3 was analyzed using the response selection ratios of the Top 2 Box and Bottom 2 Box. Regarding Questions 4 and 5, the response selection ratios of the Top 2 Box and Bottom Box were used.

2.1 Ethical considerations

Since the present study is not health-related and was conducted based on the free participation of hospital staff as part of activities to prevent disruptive behavior, ethical review based on the Ethics Committee Rules of Iwate Prefectural Central Hospital was not required. Therefore, obtaining informed consent from employees participating in the AM program was exempted.

3. Results

The group AM introductory training for all staff members was conducted 14 times in total, and the total number of participants was 1136 (attendance rate 83.2%).

The number of responses to the questionnaire on the awareness of DB inhibitory effects 1 year after the organizational AM program intervention was 730 (response rate: 54.2%) (**Figure 1**). Regarding the occupation ratio of the respondents, nurses accounted for the largest percentage (52.7%), followed by physicians (14.9%) and technicians (11.5%). There was no significant difference in the actual occupation ratio of the staff members. In terms of age group, the highest number of subjects were in their 40s (32.3%), followed by those in their 30s (27.7%) and those in their 20s (18.5%). Regarding Q1 "Do you know about AM?," the percentage of the positive response "I know about it" was 89.2% overall (n = 730) (**Figure 2**). Groupwise, the percentages for nurses (n = 385) and non-nurses (n = 345) were 91.7% and 86.4%, respectively, showing a significantly higher figure for the nurses ($p < 0.05$). Regarding Question 2 "Do you practice AM?," the percentage of the positive response of "I practice it on a regular basis" was 65.9% overall (**Figure 3**). Groupwise, the results were 71.4% and 59.8% for the nurses and non-nurses, respectively, showing a significantly higher figure for the nurses ($p < 0.001$). Regarding Question 3

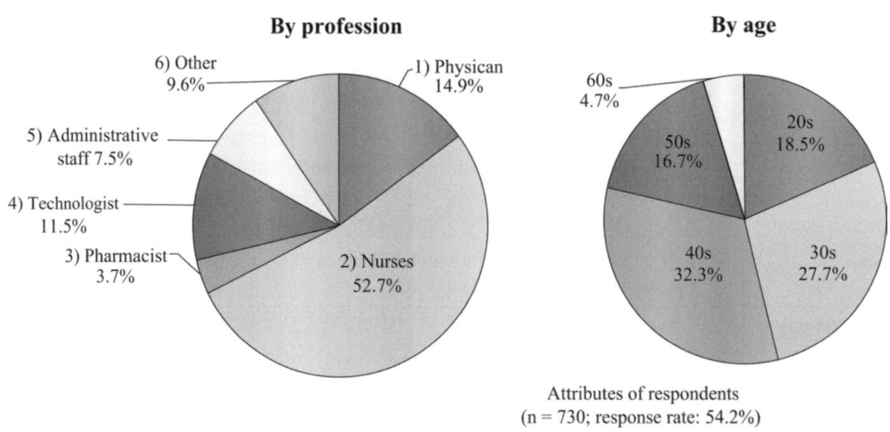

Figure 1.
Awareness survey on inhibitory effects of organizational anger management program on disruptive behavior Administered to all staff members in July 2021 (13th month after program start).

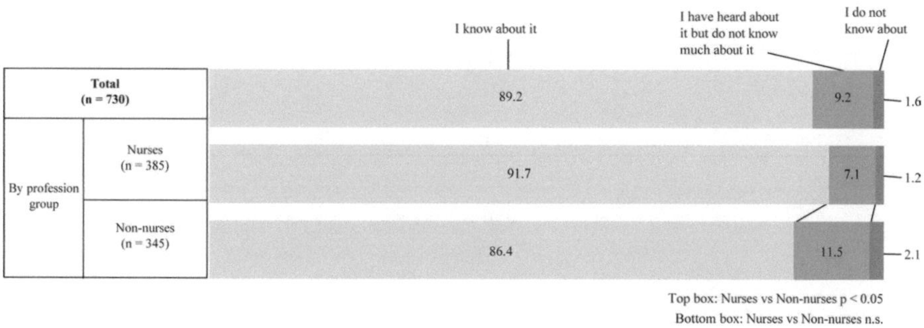

Figure 2.
Question 1 Do you know about anger management?

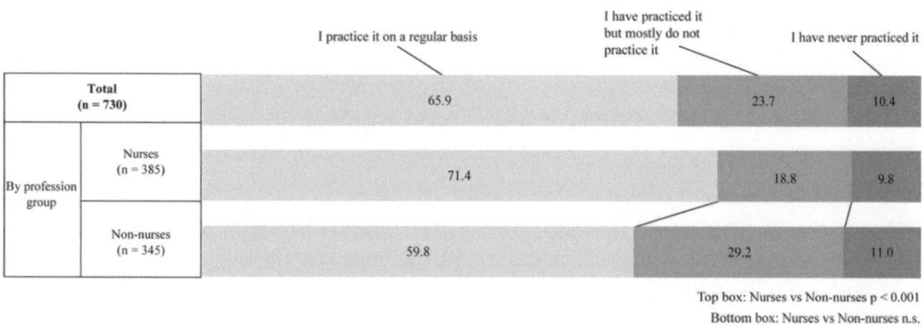

Figure 3.
Question 2 Do you practice anger management?

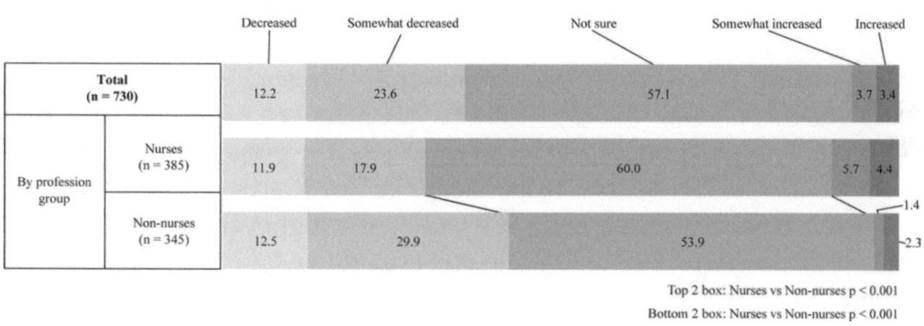

Figure 4.
Question 3 Do you think disruptive behavior in your department has diminished since the start of the organizational anger management program?

"Do you think the number of cases of DB in your department has decreased after the organizational AM program started?," the percentages of the positive responses of "Decreased" or "Somewhat Decreased" were 35.8% overall, and the percentages of negative responses of "Increased" or "Somewhat Increased" were 7.1% overall (**Figure 4**). The percentages of positive responses groupwise were 29.8% and 42.4% for the nurses and non-nurses, respectively, showing a significantly lower figure for the nurses ($p < 0.001$). The groupwise negative response rates were 10.1% and 3.7% for the nurses and non-nurses, respectively, showing a significantly higher figure for the nurses ($p < 0.001$). Regarding Question 4 "Do you think that organizational AM programs are effective in inhibiting DB?," the percentage of positive responses of "Effective" or "Somewhat Effective" was 64.2% overall, and the percentage of the

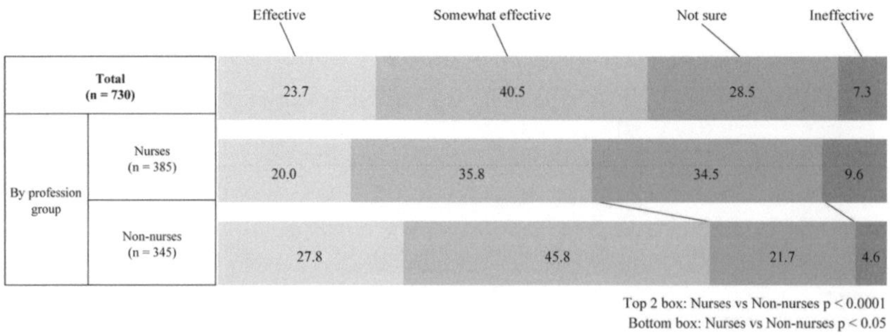

Figure 5.
Question 4 Do you think that an organizational anger management program can help control disruptive behavior?

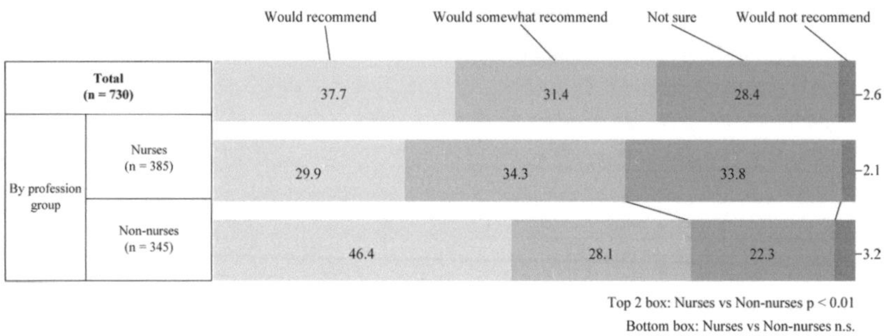

Figure 6.
Question 5 Would you recommend anger management training to your family and acquaintances?

negative response of "Ineffective" was 7.3% overall (**Figure 5**). The percentages of groupwise positive responses were 55.8% and 73.6% for the nurses and non-nurses, respectively, showing a significantly lower figure for the nurses ($p < 0.0001$). The percentages of groupwise negative responses were 9.6% and 4.6% for the nurses and non-nurses, respectively, showing a significantly higher figure for the nurses ($p < 0.05$). Regarding Question 5 "Would you recommend AM training to your family and acquaintances?," the percentage of positive responses of "Would recommend" or "Would somewhat recommend" was 69.1% overall, and the percentage of negative response of "Would not recommend" was 2.6% overall (**Figure 6**). The percentages of groupwise positive responses were 64.2% and 74.5% for the nurses and non-nurses, respectively, showing a significantly lower figure for the nurses ($p < 0.01$). In addition, in the free response (Q6) of the questionnaire, there were some opinions that the AM program had little effect on people who habitually engaged in DB (especially physicians). The respondents opined that effective initiatives aimed at such individuals are needed.

4. Discussion

DB is defined as any verbal or nonverbal behavior that harms or frightens other medical staff, patients, or family members, resulting in a reduction in the quality of patient care and a threat to patient safety [1]. While DB is known to have a significant impact on patient safety and hospital management, interventions aimed at inhibition of DB in medical institutions remain an unmet need. To the authors' knowledge, the present study is the first attempt to intervene via an organizational AM program for inhibiting DB.

Past surveys at our hospital have found that the majority of DBs (about two-thirds) are caused by feelings of anger, and it is well known that the medical field has a more complete set of factors that arouse feelings of anger than other industries. Anger among healthcare workers is often attributed to a variety of reasons, including excessive workloads, life-threatening environments where mistakes are not tolerated, family issues, relationships with colleagues, hierarchical relationships between professions, and differences in mutual values. It goes without saying that hospital organizations need to work on improving the various causes of anger, if any are addressable. However, it is clear that healthcare workers should not vent their outrage in the workplace for any reason, given the serious impact it can have on the work environment. Anger-induced DBs must be viewed as a serious threat to patient safety, quality of care, work efficiency, personal career development, and hospital operations. Therefore, we have been promoting the AM project with the aim of spreading awareness of AM throughout the organization for inhibiting DB.

The results of the questionnaire survey of all employees conducted 1 year after the start of the AM program revealed that 36% of the respondents positively regarded that the frequency of DB occurrence in their department decreased because of the AM program intervention. The percentage of respondents who positively regarded the efficacy of DB inhibition by the AM program was 64%, which was much higher than the percentage of respondents who negatively regarded it (7%). These results indicate that a notable percentage of the staff members felt that the AM program intervention was effective in inhibiting DB. Although the questionnaire response rate was somewhat low (54%), more than half of the staff members responded. Taking into consideration the fact that it was an anonymous questionnaire and that the ratio of respondents based on occupation type did not differ significantly from the actual ratio, it appears that the results of this questionnaire most likely reflected the actual feelings of the staff members regarding the number of occurrences of DB within the hospital. Based on the above findings, it cannot be ruled out that the AM program in the present study might have had some effect on DB inhibition.

The questionnaire results also revealed that the nurse group, which is generally considered to be vulnerable to DB, had a higher AM awareness and AM training practice rate in comparison with the non-nurse group; throughout the questionnaire, the percentage of positive responses regarding the DB inhibition effects of the AM program was low. The factors behind the differences in feelings between occupations regarding the efficacy of this AM program remain unknown, and further verification is needed in the future.

The organizationally introduced AM program in the present study is said to have been spontaneously born in the United States during the 1970s as a correction program for perpetrators of domestic violence and misdemeanors. Subsequently, AM was gradually systematized academically [15] and has become quite common over time [16]. At present, AM has been introduced in various workplace trainings and fields, such as adult and youth education, and its efficacy has been demonstrated [17]. Thus, AM has been established as a common method of cognitive behavioral therapy.

AM training is generally conducted individually or in groups of several individuals [18]; to date, AM has been mainly used as a correction program for physicians with habitual DB in the medical field [8, 9]. Eslamian et al. reported that they introduced an AM program on a group-by-group basis to control DB among nurses in the emergency field and achieved some results in reducing the incidence of DB [19]. However, there have been no reports of attempts by medical institutions to perform intervention through an organizational AM program with the aim of inhibiting DB. In the present study, we aimed to examine the feasibility of a cross-professional AM intervention program for all employees, with the goal of inhibiting DB by fostering a workplace culture that does not tolerate DB triggered by anger. Given that the awareness of AM is still low in Japan, it was found to be necessary to widely educate hospital staff regarding AM methods. Group AM introductory training was frequently conducted at an early stage of the activities. We additionally utilized a simple and visual method of awareness building by posting AM promotion posters. We also continued to provide motivation for AM training for each individual by sending AM-related information twice a week through groupware and broadcasts within the hospital. In the awareness survey questionnaire administered 1 year after the intervention of the AM program, 66% of the staff members responded that they practiced AM on a regular basis, showing the possibility that these continuous dissemination and simple awareness-building methods might have been effective.

The present study has several limitations. First, while the results of the present study suggested that organizational AM programs in healthcare institutions might be a somewhat effective intervention to inhibit DB, the present study was a case study in a single facility. Hence, it is difficult to generalize the obtained results. Secondly, it was extremely difficult to know the actual number of occurrences of in-hospital DB before and after the AM program intervention owing to the nature of the DB reports. It is well known that in an extremely large number of cases, the victim does not report incidents of DB owing to the fear of retaliation from the perpetrator after the DB report and because of the distrust of the hospital [7–9, 11]. Therefore, it was necessary to replace these reports with the method of evaluation using an anonymous questionnaire after the intervention of the AM program. Thus, it would be advantageous that a stable DB reporting system be established in the future. Finally, due to the nature of the study, it was necessary for the AM training to rely on the individual choice to participate by each staff member. Therefore, it was difficult to appropriately evaluate the efficacy of the AM program for the inhibition of DB. Nevertheless, despite these limitations, we believe that the present study might serve as an important resource for exploring effective intervention methods for DB inhibition in other medical institutions.

In conclusion, an organizational AM program aimed at inhibiting DB could be implemented at our facility. Although the results of the present study suggest that the AM program might be an effective method of intervention to inhibit DB, it was difficult to properly evaluate its efficacy due to the nature of the study. Furthermore, AM programs may not always be effective in the same way among different occupations; hence, further research is needed.

Acknowledgements

The authors acknowledge the business department of Iwate Prefectural Central Hospital for their cooperation in the organizational AM training and questionnaire survey. We would also like to thank Enago (**www.enago.jp**) for English language editing. This study was supported by no specific grant from any funding agency in the public, commercial, or nonprofit sectors.

Funding

The author(s) received no financial support for the research, authorship, and/or publication of this article.

Conflict of interest

The authors declare no conflicts of interests.

Author details

Hiroyuki Oura[1*] and Go Miyata[2]

1 Department of General Thoracic Surgery, Iwate Prefectural Central Hospital, Morioka, Iwate Prefecture, Japan

2 Department of Gastrointestinal Surgery, Iwate Prefectural Central Hospital, Morioka, Iwate Prefecture, Japan

*Address all correspondence to: oura_hiroyuki-prefiwate@yahoo.co.jp

References

[1] American Medical Association. Opinion E- 9.045. Physicians with Disruptive Behavior. Chicago, IL: American Medical Association; 2008

[2] Joint Commission. Behaviors that undermine a culture of safety. Sentinel Event Alert. 2008;**40**. Available from: http://www.jointcommission.org/sentinel_event_alert_issue_40_behaviors_that_undermine_a_culture_of_safety/

[3] Rosenstein AH, Russell H, Lauve R. Disruptive physician behavior contributes to nursing shortage: Study links bad behavior by doctors to nurses leaving the profession (Doctors, Nurses and Disruptive Behavior). Physician Executive. 2002;**28**(6):8-11

[4] Rosenstein AH, O'Daniel M. A survey of the impact of disruptive behaviors and communication defects on patient safety. Joint Commission Journal on Quality and Patient Safety. 2008;**34**(8):464-471

[5] Rosenstein AH. Disruptive behaviour and its impact on communication efficiency and patient care. Journal of Health Communication. 2009;**2**(4):328-340

[6] MacDonald O. Disruptive Physician Behavior. Quantia Communications, Waltham, MA: Quantia MD and the American College of Physician Executives; 2011

[7] Porto G, Lauve R. Disruptive clinician behavior: A persistent threat to patient safety. Patient safety and Quality healthcare, Lionheart Publishing, Inc. 2006;**3**:16-24. Available from: https://www.psqh.com/julaug06/disruptive.html

[8] The College of Physicians & Surgeons of Alberta. Managing disruptive behavior in the healthcare workplace. Guidance Document. Available from: https://cpsa.ca/wp-content/uploads/2021/04/Managing-Disruptive-Behavior-in-the-Healthcare-Workplace.pdf

[9] John PR, Heitt MC. Disruptive physician behavior: the importance of recognition and intervention and its impact on patient safety. Journal of Hospital Medicine. 2018;**13**(3):210-212

[10] Dunn H. Horizontal violence among nurses in the operating room. AORNJ. 2003;**78**(6):977-988

[11] Rosenstein AH, O'Daniel M. Disruptive behavior and clinical outcomes: Perceptions of nurses and physicians: Nurses, physicians, and administrators say that clinicians' disruptive behavior has negative effects on clinical outcomes. American Journal of Nursing Research. 2005;**105**(1):54-64

[12] Wilson BL, Diedrich A, Phelps CL, Choi M. Bullies at work: The impact of horizontal hostility in the hospital setting and intent to leave. The Journal of Nursing Administration. 2011;**41**(11):453-458

[13] Grissinger M. Unresolved disrespectful behavior in health care: practitioners speak up (again) - Part 1. Pharmacology & Therapeutics. 2017;**42**(1):4

[14] Rosenstein AH, Naylor B. Incidence and impact of physician and nurse disruptive behaviors in the emergency department. The Journal of Emergency Medicine. 2012;**43**(1):139-148

[15] Novaco RW. Anger Control: The Development and Evaluation of an Experimental Treatment. Lexington, Kentucky: Lexington Books; 1975

[16] Gentry WD. Anger Management for dummies. For Dummies Series (1st ed.). Hoboken, New Jersey: John Wiley & Sons; 2007

[17] Abernethy AD, Cox C. Anger management training for law enforcement personnel. Journal of Criminal Justice. 1994;**22**(5):459-466. DOI: 10.1016/0047-2352(94)90036-1

[18] Pish S, Clark-Jones T, Eschbach C, Tiret H. Anger management program participants gain behavioral changes in interpersonal relationships. Journal of Extension. 2016;**54**(5):25. Available from: https://joe.org/joe/2016october/a3.php

[19] Eslamian J, Fard SHH, Tavakol K, Yazdani M. The effect of anger management by nursing staff on violence rate against them in the emergency unit. Iranian Journal of Nursing and Midwifery Research. 2010;**15** (Suppl. 1):337-342

Chapter 3

Modern Clinical Trials in Radiation Oncology

Thomas J. FitzGerald, Fran Laurie, Matthew Iandoli, Maryann Bishop-Jodoin, Koren Smith, Kenneth Ulin, Janaki Moni, Maria Giulia Cicchetti, Stephen Kry, Michael Knopp, Ying Xiao, Mark Rosen, Fred Prior and Joel Saltz

Abstract

Clinical trials in radiation oncology have improved our translational science and patient care. All patients referred to departments of radiation oncology can be invited to participate in a clinical trial with multiple venues. Study endpoints can include intradepartmental endpoints to improve workflow and patient access as well as interdepartmental clinical translational trials that include the National Clinical Trials Network (NCTN) and industry. The quality of the trial is important to trial outcome and influences interpretation of the results of the study and how the results can be applied to patient care moving forward. Clinical trials in radiation oncology to date have accomplished much, however many important questions remain as patient care matures and systemic therapies become more sophisticated and associated with specific biomarkers and cellular expression products. In this chapter we review the history of clinical trials in radiation oncology and review the current status of the structure of quality assurance in clinical trials. We will review unanswered questions and areas to study in each disease area and how to design strategy for trials to address modern unmet needs in our discipline.

Keywords: quality, clinical trials, oncology, radiation, thoracic oncology

1. Introduction

Clinical trials have become the infrastructure for progress in both translational and clinical science in oncology. Unlike other disciplines, oncology care requires interdigitation of multiple subspecialties, each with influence on patient outcome and toxicity. As part of the National Cancer Institute (NCI) infrastructure, a robust clinical trial mechanism has been established and operational for the past 50 years. This is the National Clinical Trials Network (NCTN). Radiation oncology as a committee and discipline is incorporated into each NCTN member group and plays an important role in the structure and conduct of most trials. Radiation oncology, unlike medical oncology, can apply dose volume metrics to tumor and normal tissue and assign avoidance strategies to normal tissue. Radiation therapy (RT) is not a drug, yet colleagues in oncology care continue to apply overly simplistic thought processes to RT in the assessment of chemotherapy and RT interactions. Therefore, disease specific normal tissue constraints are written into studies to provide dose uniformity to tumor targets with protocol-specific dose volume limitations to normal tissue. This information can be transferred in digital format from anywhere in the world to a protocol quality assurance center and reviewed on a same day basis to ensure compliance with study objectives. In the next section, we will review the history of clinical trial development in radiation oncology and review the strengths and opportunities of current operational status of the quality assurance process.

2. History of quality assurance in NCTN clinical trials

By the mid 1960's, investigators and early developers of clinical trials processes sought to engage members of different institutions and participate in clinical trials. The NCI saw an advantage in further development of these processes and established a series of cooperative groups to initiate and manage clinical trials in liquid and epithelial adult oncology and pediatric oncology. Over time, this extended into discipline subspecialties including gynecologic oncology. RT began as participants within each group rapidly acquired committee status as the importance of RT in combination with systemic therapy was recognized as an important step in the development of clinical trials. Radiation oncology sections were written into protocols specifying target volume and computational techniques for quantifying dose. As the influence of radiation oncology matured, the Radiation Therapy Oncology Group (RTOG) was established as group charged with developing protocols asking RT specific questions [1–3].

In order to confirm dose was accurately delivered to the target volume intended by the study and calculated by guidelines, investigators including Arvin Glicksman and his colleague Fran Laurie designed a program to collect clinical information, planning documentation, and treatment images. The information was reviewed at the time of study completion and compliance scores were assigned and reviewed by institutional performance committees for each cooperative group [4]. Because there was a significant deviation rate on study, effort was made to move the retrospective review into an on-treatment review ideally performed during the first week on study to confirm compliance to study guidelines. The effort was performed in parallel to colleagues at the former Radiological Physics Center (RPC) who performed work using thermoluminescence dosimetry and phantoms to ensure consistent radiation dose uniformity across institutions participating in clinical trials. These efforts provided the infrastructure need to support the beginning of a quality assurance process in radiation oncology.

The former Pediatric Oncology Group (POG) established a protocol for what today would be called intermediate and early advanced stage patients with Hodgkin lymphoma, POG 8725. This study treated patients with eight cycles of hybrid chemotherapy (MOPP-ABVD alternate) with RT post chemotherapy as the point of randomization. RT was intended to be delivered to all sites of disease at presentation with dose titration permitted to areas of normal tissue tolerance including cardiac and pulmonary structures. The results of the study revealed no statistical advantage to patients receiving RT. However, a subset analysis revealed that patients treated with RT in a protocol compliant manner had a statistically significant improvement in survival at 5 years. There was a significant number of study deviations on study. Most were associated with volume of tissue treated with areas of involvement at presentation at times excluded from management due to concerns of late effects. An example of this approach would be the exclusion of involved axilla at presentation to titrate the perceived risk of a secondary event such as breast cancer in this patient study population. The overall survival in patients with study deviations was equivalent to chemotherapy alone. The survival in patients with chemotherapy and study compliant RT was 10% greater than chemotherapy alone [1–3, 5].

This study established the fact that the process of quality assurance required adjustment if radiation oncology was going to have a meaningful impact on clinical trial function and improve the conduct of clinical trials. A decision was made to have RT treatment objects, including imaging, reviewed for quality assurance purposes in order to make certain clinical trial volumes for treatment were consistent with study objectives. The protocols were Children's Oncology Group (COG) 9425 and 9426. COG 9425 was an intermediate risk study permitting mediastinal volume reduction after chemotherapy to limit dose applied to pulmonary parenchyma after five cycles of chemotherapy. COG 9426 was an early-stage protocol designed to titrate therapy based on response to induction chemotherapy. If patients were considered a rapid early responder to two cycles of chemotherapy, chemotherapy was discontinued, and the patient received 21 Gy of RT to sites of original involvement. Although at that time all materials were forwarded to quality assurance offices as hard copy, the pre-treatment review of objects considerably improved protocol compliance to RT guidelines with a statistically significant improvement in study compliance. Investigators demonstrated that the process of quality review pre-therapy could be accomplished in an enterprise manner across a clinical trial. However, the process uncovered another issue which required process improvement. COG 9426 required a response assessment after two cycles of chemotherapy. Review of response assessment was performed as a retrospective central review and what was identified was that response assessment between radiologists at the site of treatment and the central radiology reviewer was not aligned in 50% of cases. This implied that a similar process for intervention was required for radiology building upon the success for pre-treatment review for radiation oncology. The challenge became how to manage this effort in a nimble and time effective manner in order not to delay care for on-site investigators. A different approach was going to be required for data transfer in order to achieve these objectives as an enterprise function [1–3, 6].

In parallel with the effort to review objects in hard copy, colleagues in the RTOG initiated a process for digital transfer of treatment objects directly through the planning system. Jim Purdy was responsible for this fundamental change in data exchange and this process became efficient and timely for management of RT protocols [7]. The American College of Radiology Imaging Network (ACRIN) was developed and strategies for digital transfer of imaging objects directly from site investigator imaging systems to central archiving supported by the American College of Radiology (ACR) [8]. Keith White developed an internal system used by the COG based on a program he developed for digital transfer of imaging objects at his home institution to review images for tumor board. These efforts created the infrastructure required to re-visit models for data transfer and set in motion mechanisms for protocol management that remain in use today [1–3, 9–11].

The strategy for simultaneous review of imaging and RT treatment objects using digital media was applied extensively in the COG intermediate risk Hodgkin lymphoma protocol AHOD0031. In this study, adaptive therapy strategies were deployed to identify patients who had a rapid/delayed response to two cycles of chemotherapy which prompted a secondary randomization to a more titrated approach to care with rapid response and augmented care in those with a delayed response. A tertiary randomization occurred for patient with rapid early response to therapy and a complete response by imaging definition after four cycles of chemotherapy was imbedded in the study as these patients were randomized to either RT or observation. The quality assurance process for this study was extensive as more than 1700 patients were enrolled in the study requiring real time imaging response assessment at two time points in the study and pre-review of radiation oncology treatment objects. In this study metabolic and anatomic response imaging was acquired for outcome analysis. The dataset is invaluable and has been used for many publications on secondary study endpoints including but not limited to response to pleural effusions, response in bone, etc. The protocol demonstrated that these tasks assigned for managing protocols could be accomplished due in large part to the development of modern digital transfer tools and re-purposing them for management of group studies [12, 13].

Modern digital transfer tools have greatly facilitated protocol management and have brought quality assurance centers and study/site investigators together in real time on a same day basis for protocol management. Often protocols may be written in language which can be interpreted through a different prism by site investigators. The purpose of quality assurance and pre-review of objects is to ensure that the correct objects have been obtained for review in a protocol compliant format and the intended treatment plan is consistent with study objectives. The process ensures that all necessary data required for study interpretation is complete. In this manner, the dataset acquired and managed for the study is harmonized and the study results can be trusted.

The tools have also permitted expansion of clinical trial complexity including modern studies on therapy titration. These studies included surgery only for young Hodgkin lymphoma patients with highly favorable features and titration of the intended fields of RT in high-risk Hodgkin lymphoma patients to areas of less than complete response or areas that residual disease measures greater than 2.5 cm. Modern head and neck adult trials are asking titration questions for both RT target volumes and dose with patient functional endpoints to adjudicate the trial. Protocols such as this can only be successfully managed by integrative efforts of diagnostic radiology and radiation oncology as part of a central protocol review process in support of site investigators. These are important questions to answer and can only be successfully addressed in a protocol setting in order to accrue enough patients to study to answer the study question. These strategies are now applied at an enterprise level in all disease areas.

Digital transfer tools have altered the paradigm about clinical trials and how trials are managed. They have permitted real time interactions to ensure study compliance and archives for the next generation of investigators to review and ask better questions for subsequent clinical studies. The tools have also made data transfer process more nimble and given study investigators the opportunity to review all relevant imaging and RT treatment information as part of the review process. In the next section we will review pitfalls and problems associated with incomplete data acquisition.

3. Data management and problems generated by incomplete datasets

The tools today for data acquisition and management are outstanding and provide opportunity to manage protocols on a worldwide basis with real time response assessment. Other sponsor partnerships have brought quality assurance centers to standard consistent with industry needs for data compliance, security, and anonymization. These are important steps and have generated significant process improvements at quality assurance centers. This is important as many clinical trials centered in the NCTN have other sponsor partnerships imbedded into the study. The cost associated with management is largely centered in the development of the program. Once the program is established and operational, maintenance costs associated with data acquisition/management are more predictable and study driven. There is a perception, however, that cost savings is secured by data titration with ceiling imposed in the study charter to limit the amount and volume of information acquired for each study. This is an unfortunate perception and has led to limitations in the interpretation of study outcome due in part to limitations in the dataset and lack of pre-review of objects before the patient is treated on study. In the HeadSTART study of patients with locally advanced primary head and neck carcinoma evaluating in a phase III format the utility of the hypoxic cell sensitizer Tirapazamine, on-treatment review of imaging and RT treatment objects was applied for protocol management with objects to be reviewed within the first 3 days of patient treatment. Even in patients where adjustment in therapy fields were requested and adjusted for compliance, there was a statistically significant decrease in patient survival compared to patients where no adjustment was required. This would imply that every treatment mattered and created an argument that pre-treatment review of objects would be an important component to clinical trials in head and neck cancer to ensure optimal study performance [14]. The former American College of Surgeons Oncology Group Protocol Z0011intended to study the role of surgical and RT volume titration to the axilla in selected patients undergoing breast lumpectomy and post-operative RT intended to be directed to the breast only without axillary staging. It is understood that approximately 60% of the axilla including level 1 are included in the tangential RT treatment field by default as these tissues are synergistic with breast tissue. The strategy was clinically attractive as the goal was to demonstrate efficacy for more limited therapy for what was perceived as low risk patients. Targets and RT fields were not collected and completion notes describing the fields were collected for validation of what was treated to what dose. In retrospective review, however, it was found that a large number of patients with high-risk features were treated to more comprehensive regional nodal volumes than intended by the study, therefore challenging the study objectives, and making interpretation of study results more difficult as a significant number of high-risk patients were treated to extended nodal volumes. This could have been adjusted with pre-review of protocol treatment objects and conversations generated between site and study investigators ad hoc to ensure compliance objectives on study [15–17]. RTOG study 0617 became a signature study for radiation oncology as the study demonstrated non-inferiority to 60 Gy to target in comparison to 74 Gy to target. This has had significant influence in the oncology community suggesting that "less is better". What is less well known is that patient-specific diagnostic imaging defining the target was not collected as part of the quality assurance process and the plans were reviewed for quality based on submitted RT treatment objects. Although this followed more traditional quality assurance processes, for the first 3 years on study the high dose arm had statistically inferior local control compared to the low dose arm, possible implying that in the early phase of the study, tumor may have unintentionally received less dose. This may/may not have influenced trial outcome. Investigators on study accurately point out that the local control rates balanced between the two arms over time, but one has to wonder if the separation in local control did not occur in the early phase of the trial, would trial outcome have been different. The trial has become important for multiple reasons beyond target dose as the trial called attention to the importance of cardiac dose relative to long term outcome as well as provide insight into pulmonary normal tissue metrics. It is an important question to re-visit as it remains counter intuitive that a decrease in RT dose below what is applied to early-stage larynx cancer would be an advantage. The argument is toxicity, however planning techniques have improved since the initial phase of that study and it may be the right time to ask the same question with the process improvements identified in biomarker driven therapy including immunotherapy [18–22].

The data and digital objects from these trials are important and can be repurposed for multiple uses for secondary trial analysis and intercomparison of data between studies. However, each carries a flaw based on trial charter with each titrating data collection and management at different levels. The titration was well intended in order to support data management at the institutional level however titration of data can lead to unanticipated downstream consequence in outcome analysis which can shape outcome interpretation.

Therefore, trials need to be comprehensive in the data acquisition process in order to be fully confident in outcome review and use the data to answer unanticipated questions not recognized at the time of trial design. Outcome imaging is likewise crucial for study interpretation as there can be altered impressions between site and study radiology interpretation not easily recognized when we review reports. The more comprehensive we become in data acquisition, the more we can move forward in clinical trial structure. It is the responsibility of quality assurance centers, however, to ensure that the data acquisition process is not so cumbersome that it cannot be successfully managed.

4. Next steps in clinical trials

In this section progress in disease specific clinical areas is discussed and opportunities for clinical improvement in RT associated protocols is identified.

4.1 Central nervous system (CNS)

This remains an important area for clinical improvement in both adult and pediatric oncology. There is no other disease site that can affect the status of the individual afflicted with the disease from a constitutional and neuro-cognitive perspective. Brain tumors comprise 25% of childhood malignancies and primary brain tumors have a relatively equal incidence per decade in adult life, often affecting individuals during work life and family growth years. For adults with glioblastoma, recent progress has been made in the identification of biomarker expression with adjustments to care in selected patients based on genetic expression and presence of biomarkers. Studies to date have not shown a clear benefit to RT dose escalation. This may be due in part to asymmetry among radiation oncologists relative to target contours. With modern magnetic resonance (MR) imaging and sequence series, each series gives a different picture of what a target could resemble including fluid-attenuated inversion recovery (FLAIR) and single positron emission computer tomography (SPECT) imaging. Historically, most radiation oncologists generated contours from T1 images with contrast. This would identify areas of breakdown of the blood brain barrier however would not necessarily define areas of tumor deoxyribonucleic acid (DNA) synthesis which today may be defined by positron emission tomography with amino acids. There is tumor in FLAIR and when tumor is involving central structures including the corpus, SPECT may better define disease extension across the corpus which may explain failure in the contralateral hemisphere in patients with central disease when this volume is untreated. There are protocols currently active evaluating dose painting to separate target volumes using targets derived from multiple MR sequences. Establishing uniformity among radiation oncologists in this regard with agreement on dose to target will optimize the evaluation of the benefit of biomarker driven therapy moving forward as neuro-oncology is dependent on the development of therapies for the next generation of CNS clinical trials in concert with RT.

If expanded target volumes using multiple MR sequences proves to be of benefit to patients, it becomes important to the radiation oncology community to study our use of expanded targets and how they can be applied with modern image guidance moving forward. Historically, our volumetric planning language included dose to gross tumor (GTV), clinical target volume (CTV), and a planning target volume (PTV) to provide for daily patient set up variability. In selected areas an image target volume (ITV or internal gross tumor volume (IGTV)) is applied for internal motion associated with respiration. The language of expanded targets pre-dated modern image guidance. The tools of today include auto-registration of kilovoltage imaging, cone beam computer tomography, and optical tracking for positioning with motion management, therefore with more security that targets can be reproduced on a daily basis in the CNS, PTVs likely can be titrated to one-two millimeters in a manner similar to stereotactic management. This can be studied both from an intra-institutional perspective and a cooperative group perspective with online imaging and outcome imaging used to confirm the success or difficulties associated with titration of PTVs. This is important as the objective is to minimize dose to normal tissue in as safe a manner as possible and feasible. This will be important for adults and children [23].

Sub-total volume CNS directed therapy for primary and metastatic disease will become increasingly important moving forward and the radiation oncology community is assuming more responsibility for follow up in this patient population. Targeting and outcome imaging will help optimize the appropriate dose to target in selected disease areas as well as better define dose volume limitations to normal tissue.

4.2 Head and neck

Head and neck malignancies have been an important disease area for radiation oncology. With more than 30 sites of origin, significant expertise on the part of the radiation oncologist and planning team are important for optimal patient outcome. Improvements in both anatomic and metabolic imaging have improved targeting and contours for the radiation oncologist. Although contouring objects was challenging during the HeadSTART trial, metabolic imaging with PET has help to optimize the size and extent of what would be referred to as a GTV.

During the past two decades there has been an increase in the incidence of head and neck malignancies as the disease now includes viral origin as well as pre-existing environmental habits. A subset of patients with viral origin appears to have rapid early response to therapy and this cohort merits increasing attention for studies for both radiation dose and volume titration. This concept will require rigor in quality assurance to make certain that titration, especially for RT volumes, is accomplished in a uniform format. Outcome imaging is essential to perform pattern of failure analysis in order to see if radiation dose and volume can be successfully decreased in selected patients with favorable biomarkers for outcome and this should be imbedded for acquisition in clinical trials moving forward. There is evidence that immunotherapy coupled with RT can provide outcomes similar to chemotherapy and RT with a goal maintaining optimal tumor control and reduce toxicity associated with therapy. Optimizing therapy and decreasing toxicity remains important objectives moving forward, therefore clinical trials of the future will include strategies for both dose and volume titration for selected patients with more favorable features and biomarkers for a durable treatment outcome [24–29].

4.3 Thoracic oncology

Lung cancer has evolved in the past two decades. In the past, the disease was exclusively associated with environmental exposure, however recent history has demonstrated that the disease has changed both with respect to pathology and biomarker expression and targeted therapies have been approved for use with multiple subsets of patients. Immunotherapy has also become important in lung cancer and has shifted the paradigm and thought process with this disease including re-introduction of maintenance therapy.

This is important as RT remains an important co-partner to systemic therapy in this disease Because of known toxicity to pulmonary parenchyma with immunotherapy, there have been efforts in clinical trials involving thoracic RT to limit the volume of pulmonary parenchyma receiving 20 and 5 Gy as well as limit cardiac dose. Often lung tumors are located in regions vulnerable to exceeding normal tissue constraints and considerable planning skill is required to optimally treat the disease and limit dose to critical structures. Although tools for artificial intelligence used in radiation oncology strive to provide uniform dose homogeneity through the disease target, at times this is at the expense of delivering more dose to normal tissue than desired. In this circumstance, it is considered reasonable to accept more non-uniform dose distribution is less critical areas (soft tissues of the chest wall, etc.) in order to limit dose to cardio-pulmonary parenchyma. This has changed the treatment of patients on study. In order to meet cardio-pulmonary constraints defined on modern protocols, RT treatment plans are generated without elective areas to treatment which can require discontinuous planning volumes intentionally omitting areas that appear uninvolved despite target volumes contoured both inferior and superior to the volume omitted in generating the plan. The goal is to provide control of gross tumor without intentionally treating tissues as we had done on previous studies before immunotherapy and targeted therapy became available for patient care.

This is an area where motion management will play an important role moving forward. Because motion needs to be managed on-site at the participating institution in real time, it may be optimal to have institutions submit a questionnaire listing on-site equipment and complete a benchmark test demonstrating competence in contouring objects in four dimensions and making an adjustment between online imaging and planned treatment execution. Lymphoma often involves the thorax and volume modulated arc therapy provides an opportunity to be curvilinear around cardiac structures providing conformal avoidance to important structures. Cardiac avoidance may also play an important role in innate immunity for patients on study. If a significant volume of cardiac chambers is included in the treatment field, the blood pool will be exposed to therapy during the time on treatment. Lymphocytes die an intermitotic death from RT, therefore if the blood pool is exposed to radiation, a significant volume of lymphocytes will be depleted with each treatment. Clinical trials of the future will likely not contour the heart as a single structure, however tools including artificial intelligence will help contour chambers, valves, coronary arteries, and the electrical conduction system. Different disease types will influence the importance of each structure. For example, the anterior descending artery and anterior left ventricle will be important for breast cancer patients while the left atrium and electrical conduction system will be important for esophageal patients [30–38].

As outcomes improve, clinical trials will provide an opportunity to support and improve normal tissue outcome that can be quantified with RT dose volume metrics and normal tissue function.

4.4 Liver

Hepatocellular carcinoma and metastatic disease are becoming of increasing importance for patient management. The number of patients afflicted with disease in the liver is increasing and we are learning how to apply modern therapy technology to primary and secondary liver disease. One of the many challenges in modern patient care is that multiple therapies have efficacy for patients afflicted with disease including surgery, chemotherapy, stereotactic RT, and radiopharmacy. Each, however, competes for normal tissue tolerance and the benefits of multiple therapies may not be additive and may unintentionally serve to limit additional therapy due to additive toxicities. To complicate matters, at the time of diagnosis there is often pre-existing normal tissue compromise with image associated injury potentially influencing both choice and intensity of therapy. Primary hepatocellular carcinoma therapy is often optimally treated by transplant and therapies are often designed to bridge patients until transplant can be performed. Often, however, patients are not candidates for transplant, and they need to be managed medically with either stereotactic RT or radiopharmacy including modern targeted therapy. The choice of therapy can be nuanced and driven by the heath of the patient and liver function including Child-Pugh status. Therapies, although available for patient care, need to be studied in more detail to know how to apply them and limit risk of injury. Although radiopharmacy with Yttrium-90 (Y-90) can deliver dose to target, there are clinical challenges associated with the delivery of therapy. Although intrahepatic catheters can be accurately placed, tumor vascularity is irregular with areas of limited vascular access, therefore shunt and movement of particles/dose away from the intended target can result in dose delivery to unintended target and limited dose to the intended target. Because of the previous lack of computational software for post therapy dosimetry, quality assurance metrics have been limited to the activity of the isotope. Today, computational dosimetry software is now available to assess dose to tumor target and normal tissue using SPECT as an imaging tool to perform voxel dosimetry. This will help move the care of these patients to a more optimal assessment of dose to volume and assess, especially with Y-90, in defining areas receiving less than tumor specific dose and which areas require additional dose augmentation. Although Y-90 is thought to be specific to target, there can be unintended consequence to uninvolved segments of hepatic parenchyma through migration and dose can extend to organs abutting hepatic parenchyma including renal parenchyma and bowel. Modern radiosurgery can place limitations and dose gradients in a secure manner across targets with motion management and image validation [39–45].

There is a paucity of studies comparing therapies which serves to limit advancing the discussion concerning safety and efficacy of each approach. Often patient care is driven by the specific expertise of providers on-site. Each case will have tumor specific vascularity, location, and size, therefore, randomized clinical trials will be difficult to perform in this area. A registry with clinical information, therapy imaging/dosimetry, and outcome imaging may be the best initial approach to developing a definition of dose volume metrics for patient safety.

4.5 Gastrointestinal

Gastrointestinal (GI) disease encompasses many important areas for radiation oncology. Esophageal cancer is highly responsive to chemoradiotherapy, and pre-operative therapy has rapidly become the standard of care. The targets for RT are driven in large part by imaging generated from positron emission tomography and endoscopy. Initial studies using image-guided definitions for targeting applied generous superior and inferior margins, however extended volume therapy into uninvolved nodal regions can make planning difficult to meet dose volume constraints especially for cardiac and pulmonary parenchyma. This merits further investigation as can targets be titrated considering cardiac and pulmonary parenchyma as "natural barriers" even though they abut tumor targets. In other words, can the gross tumor volume and the CTV be synergistic in this location with the image-guided target symbiotic with the PTV. Outcome metrics relative to cardiac and pulmonary parenchyma balanced with outcome imaging to identify local regional failure could be part of radiation oncology study objectives challenging traditional computational metrics and tumor target definition balanced with normal tissue tolerance metrics [46, 47].

A similar approach can be applied for pancreatic cancer. Although RT has been lateralized in clinical protocol development, meta-analysis continues to suggest an important role for RT in this disease. Protracted chemotherapy protocols with RT applied at the time of disease progression limits the perceived effectiveness of RT given as either definitive therapy or post-operative therapy. However, therapy must be balanced with normal tissue tolerance as hepatic, renal, and bowel volumes must be respected including important anastomoses in post-operative patients. RT will eventually be seen again as an asset in this disease and radiation committees will be cognizant of the responsibility we need to apply to this situation particularly in patients with borderline resectable disease [48].

There is increasing information that compressed fractionation strategies can be applied to patients with rectal cancer. Short term data suggests that compressed schedules are non-inferior with respect to surgical intervention with variability in contouring structures including the mesorectum. More long-term data is needed to determine if compressed schedules are non-inferior to local control and normal tissue function. This is an area where tissue is available both pre and post therapy and biomarkers may play a role in outcome assessment [49, 50].

Anal cancers remain of increasing importance in the treatment community. Protocols have often applied a uniform strategy to patients with varied stage and tumor burden. Moving forward, stratification of patients in clinical trials by stage/tumor burden including RT alone trials in selected favorable patients will be an important next step in management. Likewise, we need to define as best as possible what target volumes should resemble for modern patient care. For example, can the mesorectum be considered a CTV at risk with the tumor defined on positron emission tomography as the CTV of high risk? If so, dose painting can be applied including optimal definition of what nodal volumes are at risk. Only clinical trials with shared data information can answer these important questions [51].

4.6 Genitourinary

Genitourinary (GU) oncology remains an important area of research for radiation oncology. Prostate cancer is exceptionally well treated with modern radiation oncology. With image guidance and intensity modulation, outcomes have been exceptional and continue to improve. Because in large part to limited dose to normal tissue including bladder and rectum, compressed fractionation schedules have become more popular in clinical care. It is important to couple these changes with patient symptoms at presentation in order to optimize dose and fractionation schemes to pre-existing genitourinary health. Clinical trials will help us segregate which patients are more optimally served with traditional fractionation likely including those with high-risk features including the need for regional therapy. Oligometastasis therapy is moving forward at a rapid pace as outcome appears to be improved with more aggressive management upfront in patients with limited metastatic disease. The nature of treatment in this situation coupled with emerging technologies including radiopharmacy hold promise to improve survival in this patient cohort. It will be important to include modern anatomic and metabolic imaging as part of staging. This will help optimize targets of therapy and identify patients in need of extended volume therapy due to oligometastatic disease [52–55].

One potential area for clinical trials is to think of the prostate differently with respect to target technology. Today we think of the prostate gland as a uniform structure for target definition, often independent of disease identified on imaging including MR. As imaging improves, can we consider the gland as a target volume of intermediate risk and dose paint image associated areas of concern as targets of high risk. This would potentially further serve to titrate dose across critical structures including bladder, urethra, nerve bundles, and rectum potentially improving normal tissue outcome and not sacrifice local control.

Bladder preservation technology is improving. Often these patients are medically vulnerable, therefore therapy choices are often influenced by medical co-morbidities. Likewise, the choice for systemic therapy in combination with RT has to recognize the potential for toxicity, therefore choices are balanced. Immunotherapy coupled with RT remains under investigation and appears well tolerate. These pathways will need further exploration [56].

Aggressive RT management upfront of renal metastasis will also be important to study moving forward as this may make response to targeted and immunotherapies more durable and not interrupt systemic therapy treatment schedule.

4.7 Gynecologic

This remains an important area to study as gynecologic malignancies remain an important worldwide public health issue. The incidence of cervix cancer worldwide including medically underserved populations continues to grow and often patients with limited access to care present with advanced stage disease. Modern imaging including positron emission tomography has demonstrated an increase incidence of nodal involvement at presentation than was previously acknowledged. Treatment programs with RT coupled with brachytherapy remain important and essential to patient care, however improving outcome will require optimal application of new and novel systemic therapy. Biomarker-driven clinical trials including immunotherapy will be important to see if outcome can be improved in these patients [55–61].

Although endometrial cancers are often found early in the disease process because of clinical symptoms, selected patients do not uniformly have optimal outcomes and these patients become candidates for chemotherapy and biomarker-driven therapy coupled with surgery and RT to optimize tumor control. These can include carcinosarcoma and papillary serous histology [62–64]. Current protocols seek to define improvements in systemic care. With biomarker-driven care and immunotherapy, protocols for therapy are evaluating these issues. Medically inoperable patients are increasing in frequency as society ages, therefore protocols optimizing care for these patients is likewise important moving forward. Ovarian carcinoma remains a clinical challenge as to date, imaging of disease has not been optimal however improvements in imaging are anticipated. Biomarker-driven therapeutic options are important moving forward to optimize care for this cohort and well as those with primary peritoneal disease.

4.8 Musculoskeletal

For both adults and pediatric patients, this is an area of increasing importance. For adults, patients are often treated with pre-operative RT in order to facilitate surgical resection. This provides opportunities to use pre and post therapy imaging to determine if radiomics predicts for response and outcome. Tissue is available both pre and post therapy, therefore elements of tumor microenvironment and tumor related biomarkers are available for study. Tumor specific biomarkers identified in post therapy specimens may provide insight into resistance molecules and mechanisms for the next generation of studies and identify additional agents and biomarker driven therapy could be applied on a pre-operative basis [65, 66].

For childhood sarcoma, these diseases affect both bone and soft tissue. Pediatric tumors are less likely to be influenced by epigenetics. In the NCI pediatric Molecular Analysis for Therapy Choice (MATCH) trial, a significant percentage of pediatric tumors have an actionable mutation. These diseases have remarkable responses to systemic therapy and often local control can be achieved with surgical and RT titration of resection and RT dose. These have been studied by outstanding investigators in the past within cooperative group disease specific committees. The structure provided by the committees will be an excellent resource moving forward as systemic therapy and personalized application of targeted therapy moves forward. There will be an increasing use of particle therapy for these diseases in order to exclude normal tissue from the RT treatment field and decrease sequelae from management [67].

4.9 Pediatrics

Process improvements in the technology of RT will significantly benefit pediatric radiation oncology. The increasing use of particles and intensity modulation coupled with image guidance will limit dose to unintended structures and serve to further improve outcome relative to tumor control and normal tissue. This will be important in all areas of pediatric oncology including the aforementioned sarcoma subgroups but also for pediatric brain tumors and all additional disease areas. Because of the security provided in treatment reproducibility, PTVs can be titrated to institutional tolerance. These is especially important in younger children as an additional 1–2 mm of expansion can significantly influence the volume of normal tissue receiving full dose, therefore when feasible, titrating high dose and low dose volumes can have a measurable impact on outcome. This is true in all disease areas [68–74].

5. Conclusions

RT has matured as a discipline with tools now readily available to generate metrics to assess both tumor control and normal tissue outcome. Databases are available to house information in a format to re-purpose the data generated from RT treatment objects and imaging to perform accurate and believable outcome assessment. The Cancer Imaging Archive (TCIA) has been developed to house data in a format available for clinical/translational research. Data acquisition and management processes are robust and prepared to function at an enterprise level to move us forward [20, 75].

Author details

Thomas J. FitzGerald[1*], Fran Laurie[1], Matthew Iandoli[1], Maryann Bishop-Jodoin[1], Koren Smith[1], Kenneth Ulin[1], Janaki Moni[1], Maria Giulia Cicchetti[1], Stephen Kry[2], Michael Knopp[3], Ying Xiao[4], Mark Rosen[5], Fred Prior[6] and Joel Saltz[7]

1 Imaging and Radiation Oncology Core-RI, Department of Radiation Oncology, UMass Chan Medical School, Lincoln, USA

2 Imaging and Radiation Oncology Core-Houston, Division of Radiation Oncology, MD Anderson, Houston, USA

3 Imaging and Radiation Oncology Core-Ohio, Department of Radiology, The Ohio State University, Columbus, USA

4 Imaging and Radiation Oncology Core Philadelphia, Department of Radiation Oncology, University of Pennsylvania, Philadelphia, USA

5 Imaging and Radiation Oncology Core Philadelphia, Department of Radiology, University of Pennsylvania, Philadelphia, USA

6 Department of Biomedical Informatics, University of Arkansas, Little Rock, USA

7 Department of Biomedical Informatics, Stony Brook University, Stony Brook, USA

*Address all correspondence to: tj.fitzgerald@umassmemorial.org

References

[1] FitzGerald TJ, Urie M, Ulin K, Laurie F, Yorty J, Hanusik R, et al. Processes for quality improvements in radiation oncology clinical trials. International Journal of Radiation Oncology, Biology, Physics. 2008;**71**(1S):S76-S79

[2] FitzGerald TJ, Bishop-Jodoin M, Followill DS, Galvin J, Knopp MV, Michalski JM, et al. Imaging and data acquisition in clinical trials for radiation therapy. International Journal of Radiation Oncology, Biology, Physics. 2016;**94**(2):404-411

[3] Fitzgerald TJ, Bishop-Jodoin M, Bosch WR, Curran WJ, Followill DS, Galvin JM, et al. Future vision for the quality assurance of oncology clinical trials. Frontiers in Oncology. 2013;**3**:31

[4] Arvin S. Glicksman, MD 1924 to 2020. Practical Radiation Oncology. 2020;**10**(5):301-303

[5] Weiner MA, Leventhal B, Brecher ML, Marcus RB, Cantor A, Gieser PW, et al. Randomized study of intensive MOPP-ABVD with or without low-dose total-nodal radiation therapy in the treatment of stages IIb, IIIa2, IIIb, and IV Hodgkin's disease in pediatric patients: A Pediatric Oncology Group study. Journal of Clinical Oncology. 1997;**15**(8):2769-2779

[6] Eich HT, Engenhart-Cabillic R, Hansemann K, Lukas P, Schneeweiss A, Seegenschmiedt H, et al. Quality control of involved field radiotherapy in patients with early-favorable (HD10) and early-unfavorable (HD11) Hodgkin's lymphoma: An analysis of the German Hodgkin study group. International Journal of Radiation Oncology, Biology, Physics. 2008;**71**(5):1419-1424

[7] Purdy JA. Quality assurance issues in conducting multi-institutional advanced technology clinical trials. International Journal of Radiation Oncology, Biology, Physics. 2008;**71**(1S):S66-S70

[8] Giaddui T, Yu J, Manfredi D, Linnemann N, Hunter J, O'Meara E, et al. Structures' validation profiles in transmission of imaging and data (TRIAD) for automated National Clinical Trials Network (NCTN) clinical trial digital data quality assurance. Practical Radiation Oncology. 2016;**6**(5):331-333

[9] Weber DC, Tomsej M, Melidis C, Hurkmans CW. QA makes a clinical trial stronger: Evidence-based medicine in radiation therapy. Radiotherapy and Oncology. 2012;**105**(1):4-8

[10] Ohri N, Shen X, Dicker AP, Doyle LA, Harrison AS, Showalter TN. Radiotherapy protocol deviations and clinical outcomes: A meta-analysis of cooperative group clinical trials. Journal of the National Cancer Institute. 2013;**105**(6):387-393

[11] Fairchild A, Straube W, Laurie F, Followill D. Does quality of radiation therapy predict outcomes of multicenter cooperative group trials? A literature review. International Journal of Radiation Oncology, Biology, Physics. 2013;**87**(2):246-260

[12] Friedman DL, Chen L, Wolden S, Buxton A, McCarten K, FitzGerald TJ, et al. Dose-intensive response-based chemotherapy and radiation therapy for children and adolescents with newly diagnosed intermediate-risk Hodgkin lymphoma: A report from the Children's oncology group study AHOD0031. Journal of Clinical Oncology. 2014;**32**(32):3651-3658

[13] Dharmarajan KV, Friedman DL, FitzGerald TJ, McCarten KM, Constine LS, Chen L, et al. Radiotherapy quality assurance report from Children's oncology group AHOD0031. International Journal of Radiation Oncology, Biology, Physics. 2015;**91**(5):1065-1071

[14] Peters LJ, O'Sullivan B, Giralt J, Fitzgerald TJ, Trotti A, Bernier J, et al. Critical impact of radiotherapy protocol compliance and quality in the treatment of advanced head and neck cancer: Results from TROG 02.02. Journal of Clinical Oncology. 2010;**28**(18):2996-3001

[15] Giuliano AE, Ballman KV, McCall L, Beitsch PD, Brennan MB, Kelemen PR, et al. Effect of axillary dissection vs no axillary dissection on 10-year overall survival among women with invasive breast cancer and sentinel node metastasis: The ACOSOG Z0011 (Alliance) randomized clinical trial. Journal of the American Medical Association. 2017;**318**(10):918-926

[16] Jagsi R, Chadha M, Moni J, Ballman K, Laurie F, Buchholz TA, et al. Radiation field design in the ACOSOG Z0011 (Alliance) trial. Journal of Clinical Oncology. 2014;**32**(32):3600-3606

[17] Reznik J, Cicchetti MG, Degaspe B, Fitzgerald TJ. Analysis of axillary coverage during tangential radiation therapy to the breast. International Journal of Radiation Oncology, Biology, Physics. 2005;**61**(1):163-168

[18] Buckler AJ, Boellaard R. Standardization of quantitative imaging: The time is right, and 18F-FDG PET/CT is a good place to start. Journal of Nuclear Medicine. 2011;**52**(2):171-172

[19] Curran S, Muellner A, Schwartz LH. Imaging response assessment in oncology. Cancer Imaging. 2006;**6**:S126-S130

[20] Saltz J, Almeida J, Gao Y, Sharma A, Bremer E, DiPrima T, et al. Towards generation, management, and exploration of combined radiomics and pathomics datasets for cancer research. AMIA Summits on Translational Science Proceedings. 2017;**2017**:85-94

[21] Gillies RJ, Kinahan PE, Hricak H. Radiomics: Images are more than pictures, they are data. Radiology. 2016;**278**(2):563-577

[22] Wolchok JD, Hoos A, O'Day S, Weber JS, Hamid O, Lebbé C, et al. Guidelines for the evaluation of immune therapy activity in solid tumors: Immune-related response criteria. Clinical Cancer Research. 2009;**15**(23):7412-7420

[23] Kruser TJ, Bosch WR, Badiyan SN, Bovi JA, Ghia AJ, Kim MM, et al. NRG brain tumor specialists consensus guidelines for glioblastoma contouring. Journal of Neuro-Oncology. 2019;**143**(1):157-166

[24] Grégoire V, Eisbruch A, Hamoir M, Levendag P. Proposal for the delineation of the nodal CTV in the node-positive and the post-operative neck. Radiotherapy and Oncology. 2006;**79**(1):15-20

[25] Grégoire V, Ang K, Budach W, Grau C, Hamoir M, Langendijk JA, et al. Delineation of the neck node levels for head and neck tumors: A 2013 update. DAHANCA, EORTC, HKNPCSG, NCIC CTG, NCRI, RTOG, TROG consensus guidelines. Radiotherapy and Oncology. 2014;**110**(1):172-181

[26] Biau J, Lapeyre M, Troussier I, Budach W, Giralt J, Grau C, et al. Selection of lymph node target volumes

for definitive head and neck radiation therapy: A 2019 update. Radiotherapy and Oncology. 2019;**134**:1-9

[27] Rasch CR, Steenbakkers RJ, Fitton I, Duppen JC, Nowak PJ, Pameijer FA, et al. Decreased 3D observer variation with matched CT-MRI, for target delineation in nasopharynx cancer. Radiation Oncology. 2010;**5**:21

[28] van der Veen J, Gulyban A, Nuyts S. Interobserver variability in delineation of target volumes in head and neck cancer. Radiotherapy and Oncology. 2019;**137**:9-15

[29] Nelms BE, Tomé WA, Robinson G, Wheeler J. Variations in the contouring of organs at risk: Test case from a patient with oropharyngeal cancer. International Journal of Radiation Oncology. 2012;**82**(1):368-378

[30] Brahmer J, Reckamp KL, Baas P, Crinò L, Eberhardt WE, Poddubskaya E, et al. Nivolumab versus docetaxel in advanced squamous-cell non-small-cell lung cancer. The New England Journal of Medicine. 2015;**373**(2):123-135

[31] Borghaei H, Paz-Ares L, Horn L, Spigel DR, Steins M, Ready NE, et al. Nivolumab versus docetaxel in advanced nonsquamous non-small-cell lung cancer. The New England Journal of Medicine. 2015;**373**(17):1627-1639

[32] Antonia SJ, Villegas A, Daniel D, Vicente D, Murakami S, Hui R, et al. Durvalumab after chemoradiotherapy in stage III non-small-cell lung cancer. The New England Journal of Medicine. 2017;**377**(20):1919-1929

[33] Simone CB 2nd, Burri SH, Heinzerling JH. Novel radiotherapy approaches for lung cancer: Combining radiation therapy with targeted and immunotherapies. Translational Lung Cancer Research. 2015;**4**:545-552

[34] Simone CB 2nd, Berman AT, Jabbour SK. Harnessing the potential synergy of combining radiation therapy and immunotherapy for thoracic malignancies. Translational Lung Cancer Research. 2017;**6**:109-112

[35] Deng L, Liang H, Burnette B, Beckett M, Darga T, Weichselbaum RR, et al. Irradiation and anti-PD-L1 treatment synergistically promote antitumor immunity in mice. The Journal of Clinical Investigation. 2014;**124**(2):687-695

[36] Simone CB 2nd, Houshmand S, Kalbasi A, Salavati A, Alavi A. PET-based thoracic radiation oncology. PET Clinics. 2016;**11**(3):319-332

[37] Verma V, Choi JI, Sawant A, Gullapalli RP, Chen W, Alavi A, et al. Use of PET and other functional imaging to guide target delineation in radiation oncology. Seminars in Radiation Oncology. 2018;**28**(3):171-177

[38] Soon YY, Chen D, Tan TH, Seong Tey JC. Quality of reporting on thoracic radiotherapy technique in prospective lung cancer trials: A systematic review. Medicine (Baltimore). 2019;**98**(26):e16124

[39] European Association for the Study of the Liver. EASL clinical practice guidelines: Management of hepatocellular carcinoma. Journal of Hepatology. 2018;**69**(1):182-236

[40] Rim CH, Seong J. Application of radiotherapy for hepatocellular carcinoma in current clinical practice guidelines. Radiation Oncology Journal. 2016;**34**(3):160-167

[41] Rim CH, Kim CY, Yang DS, Yoon WS. Comparison of radiation therapy modalities for hepatocellular carcinoma with portal vein thrombosis:

A meta-analysis and systematic review. Radiotherapy and Oncology. 2018;**129**(1):112-122

[42] Rim CH, Kim CY, Yang DS, Yoon WS. External beam radiation therapy to hepatocellular carcinoma involving inferior vena cava and/or right atrium: A meta-analysis and systemic review. Radiotherapy and Oncology. 2018;**129**(1):123-129

[43] Chow PK, Choo SP, Ng DC, Lo RH, Wang ML, Toh HC, et al. National Cancer Centre Singapore Consensus Guidelines for hepatocellular carcinoma. Liver Cancer. 2016;**5**(2):97-106

[44] Rim CH, Kim HJ, Seong J. Clinical feasibility and efficacy of stereotactic body radiotherapy for hepatocellular carcinoma: A systematic review and meta-analysis of observational studies. Radiotherapy and Oncology. 2019;**131**:135-144

[45] Rim CH, Kim CY, Yang DS, Yoon WS. The role of external beam radiotherapy for hepatocellular carcinoma patients with lymph node metastasis: A meta-analysis of observational studies. Cancer Management and Research. 2018;**10**:3305-3315

[46] Boustani J, Rivin Del Campo E, Blanc J, Peiffert D, Benezery K, Pereira R, et al. Quality assurance of dose-escalated radiation therapy in a randomized trial for locally advanced oesophageal cancer. International Journal of Radiation Oncology, Biology, Physics. 2019;**105**(2):329-337

[47] Bolger JC, Donohoe CL, Lowery M, Reynolds JV. Advances in the curative management of oesophageal cancer. British Journal of Cancer. 2022;**126**(5):706-717

[48] Huguet F, Goodman KA, Azria D, Racadot S, Abrams RA. Radiotherapy technical considerations in the management of locally advanced pancreatic cancer: American-French consensus recommendations. International Journal of Radiation Oncology, Biology, Physics. 2012;**83**(5):1355-1364

[49] van den Ende RPJ, Peters FP, Harderwijk E, Rütten H, Bouwmans L, Berbee M, et al. Radiotherapy quality assurance for mesorectum treatment planning within the multi-center phase II STAR-TReC trial: Dutch results. Radiation Oncology. 2020;**15**(1):41

[50] Wo JY, Anker CJ, Ashman JB, Bhadkamkar NA, Bradfield L, Chang DT, et al. Radiation therapy for rectal Cancer: Executive summary of an ASTRO clinical practice guideline. Practical Radiation Oncology. 2021;**11**(1):13-25

[51] Benson AB, Venook AP, Al-Hawary MM, Cederquist L, Chen YJ, Ciombor KK, et al. Anal carcinoma, version 2.2018, NCCN clinical practice guidelines in oncology. Journal of the National Comprehensive Cancer Network. 2018;**16**(7):852-871

[52] Achard V, Jaccard M, Vanhoutte F, Siva S, Heikkilä R, Dirix P, et al. Oligorecurrent nodal prostate cancer: Radiotherapy quality assurance of the randomized PEACE V-STORM phase II trial. Radiotherapy and Oncology. 2022;**172**:1-9

[53] Lawton CA, Michalski J, El-Naqa I, Buyyounouski MK, Lee WR, Menard C, et al. RTOG GU radiation oncology specialists reach consensus on pelvic lymph node volumes for high-risk prostate cancer. International Journal of Radiation Oncology, Biology, Physics. 2009;**74**(2):383-387

[54] Hall WA, Paulson E, Davis BJ, Spratt DE, Morgan TM, Dearnaley D,

et al. NRG oncology updated international consensus atlas on pelvic lymph node volumes for intact and postoperative prostate Cancer. International Journal of Radiation Oncology, Biology, Physics. 2021;**109**(1):174-185

[55] Sarwar R, Altaf S, Khan RMA, Buzdar SA, Iqbal K. VMAT treatment plan acceptability and quality assurance study for prostate cancer in radiotherapy. Journal of Radiotherapy in Practice. 2020;**20**(1):43-48

[56] Patel E, Tsang Y, Baker A, Callender J, Hafeez S, Hall E, et al. Quality assuring "plan of the day" selection in a multicentre adaptive bladder trial: Implementation of a pre-accrual IGRT guidance and assessment module. Clinical and Translational Radiation Oncology. 2019;**19**:27-32

[57] Kasuya G, Toita T, Furutani K, Kodaira T, Ohno T, Kaneyasu Y, et al. Distribution patterns of metastatic pelvic lymph nodes assessed by CT/MRI in patients with uterine cervical cancer. Radiation Oncology. 2013;**8**:139

[58] Hwang L, Bailey A, Lea J, Albuquerque K. Para-aortic nodal metastases in cervical cancer: A blind spot in the International Federation of Gynecology and Obstetrics staging system: Current diagnosis and management. Future Oncology. 2015;**11**(2):309-322

[59] Bats AS, Mathevet P, Buenerd A, Orliaguet I, Mery E, Zerdoud S, et al. The sentinel node technique detects unexpected drainage pathways and allows nodal ultrastaging in early cervical cancer: Insights from the multicenter prospective SENTICOL study. Annals of Surgical Oncology. 2013;**20**(2):413-422

[60] Bailey A, Hwang L, Xi Y, McKeever M, Albuquerque K. CT mapping of metastatic nodal disease in patients with advanced cervical cancer in an indigent US population: Implications for resource ctilization and conformal radiation (CRT) planning. In: 2014 Scientific Assembly and Annual Meeting. Chicago IL: Radiological Society of North America (RSNA); 2014. Available from: http://archive.rsna.org/2014/14013248.html. [Accessed: August 1, 2022]

[61] Toita T, Kato S, Ishikura S, Tsujino K, Kodaira T, Uno T, et al. Radiotherapy quality assurance of the Japanese Gynecologic oncology group study (JGOG1066): A cooperative phase II study of concurrent chemoradiotherapy for uterine cervical cancer. International Journal of Clinical Oncology. 2011;**16**(4):379-386

[62] Jhingran A, Winter K, Portelance L, Miller B, Salehpour M, Gaur R, et al. A phase II study of intensity modulated radiation therapy to the pelvis for postoperative patients with endometrial carcinoma: Radiation therapy oncology group trial 0418. International Journal of Radiation Oncology, Biology, Physics. 2012;**84**(1):e23-e28

[63] Wortman BG, Astreinidou E, Laman MS, van der Steen-Banasik EM, Lutgens LCHW, Westerveld H, et al. Brachytherapy quality assurance in the PORTEC-4a trial for molecular-integrated risk profile guided adjuvant treatment of endometrial cancer. Radiotherapy and Oncology. 2021;**155**:160-166

[64] Harkenrider MM, Block AM, Siddiqui ZA, Small W Jr. The role of vaginal cuff brachytherapy in endometrial cancer. Gynecologic Oncology. 2015;**136**(2):365-372

[65] Salerno KE, Alektiar KM, Baldini EH, Bedi M, Bishop AJ, Bradfield L, et al. Radiation therapy for treatment of

soft tissue sarcoma in adults: Executive summary of an ASTRO clinical practice guideline. Practical Radiation Oncology. 2021;**11**(5):339-351

[66] Beane JD, Yang JC, White D, Steinberg SM, Rosenberg SA, Rudloff U. Efficacy of adjuvant radiation therapy in the treatment of soft tissue sarcoma of the extremity: 20-year follow-up of a randomized prospective trial. Annals of Surgical Oncology. 2014;**21**(8):2484-2489

[67] Breneman JC, Donaldson SS, Constine L, Merchant T, Marcus K, Paulino AC, et al. The Children's oncology group radiation oncology discipline: 15 years of contributions to the treatment of childhood cancer. International Journal of Radiation Oncology, Biology, Physics. 2018;**101**(4):860-874

[68] Michalski JM, Janss A, Vezina G, Gajjar A, Pollack I, Merchant TE, et al. Results of COG ACNS0331: A phase III trial of involved-field radiotherapy (IFRT) and low dose craniospinal irradiation (LD-CSI) with chemotherapy in average-risk medulloblastoma: A report from the Children's oncology group. International Journal of Radiation Oncology, Biology, Physics. 2016;**96**(5):937-938

[69] Wolden S. Quality Assurance in Rhabdomyosarcoma within COG. Ljubljana, Slovenia: Paediatric Radiation Oncology Society (PROS); 2015

[70] Packer RJ, Gajjar A, Vezina G, Rorke-Adams L, Burger PC, Robertson PL, et al. Phase III study of craniospinal radiation therapy followed by adjuvant chemotherapy for newly diagnosed average-risk medulloblastoma. Journal of Clinical Oncology. 2006;**24**(25):4202-4208

[71] Parzuchowski A, Bush R, Pei Q, Friedman DL, FitzGerald TJ, Wolden SL, et al. Patterns of involved-field radiation therapy protocol deviations in pediatric versus adolescent and young adults with Hodgkin lymphoma: A report from the Children's oncology group AHOD0031. International Journal of Radiation Oncology, Biology, Physics. 2018;**100**(5):1119-1125

[72] Gaze MN, Boterberg T, Dieckmann K, Hörmann M, Gains JE, Sullivan KP, et al. Results of a quality assurance review of external beam radiation therapy in the International Society of Paediatric Oncology (Europe) neuroblastoma Group's high-risk neuroblastoma trial: A SIOPEN study. International Journal of Radiation Oncology, Biology, Physics. 2013;**85**(1):170-174

[73] Gains JE, Stacey C, Rosenberg I, Mandeville HC, Chang YC, D'Souza D, et al. Intensity-modulated arc therapy to improve radiation dose delivery in the treatment of abdominal neuroblastoma. Future Oncology. 2013;**9**(3):439-449

[74] Carrie C, Hoffstetter S, Gomez F, Moncho V, Doz F, Alapetite C, et al. Impact of targeting deviations on outcome in medulloblastoma: Study of the French Society of Pediatric Oncology (SFOP). International Journal of Radiation Oncology, Biology, Physics. 1999;**45**(2):435-439

[75] Prior F, Smith K, Sharma A, Kirby J, Tarbox L, Clark K, et al. The public cancer radiology imaging collections of the Cancer imaging archive. Scientific Data. 2017;**4**:170124

Chapter 4

Hospital Ethical Climate and Its Influence on Clinical Nurses' Perception on Their Organizational Citizenship Performance

Teketel Ermias Geltore

Abstract

Healthcare development mainly depends on nurses' activities, since nurses often take much time in contacting patients during clinical activities. Their awareness of the hospital's moral climate disturbs nurses' attitudes and associated ethical concerns. Hospital ethical climates have become a crucial working area element for nurses to prepare and apply ethical judgments. The ethical climate is one feature of an institution that denotes the collective insights of morally correct activities and techniques of handling ethically varied conduct. Better consciousness of the difficulty of ethical problems in the health facility situation has powered attention to nursing ethics. Yet, there is insufficient data on the connection between nurses' awareness of the ethical climate worldwide. Hospital ethical climate has been studied in several industrial countries for decades but has only been investigated in some developing countries in the past two decades. In general, the chapter explained the perception of nurses and correlation between hospital ethical climate and job satisfaction, and dimensions of job design.

Keywords: ethical climates, nurses, ethics, hospital, nursing, profession

1. Introduction

Nurses making the biggest group of experts in the healthcare delivery system, who communicate broadly with patients. They are well-thought-out and a backbone of the healthcare system in terms of provision of the quality of services to patients. Thus, it is significant for nurses to have a great sense of welfare and success in the face of recent encounters and difficulties [1, 2].

Employees are the fundamental asset of health-care facilities. Nurses are the chief human resources in healthcare organizations, who play a pivotal role in providing unceasing great quality care [3]. Ethical climate denotes the collective views of ethically correct conduct and way of treating ethically deviated actions [4]. Organizational climate is defined as the recurring patterns of behavior and feelings that describe life in the organization that is more linked to atmosphere and values [5, 6].

Every day, when nurses perform their daily activities, they face different types of problems and issues that might be unpredictable with their perceptions. Due to clinical diagnosis and treatments, nurses have repeated ethical concerns with patients, attendants, and other staffs. For instance, because the staff number of nurses is inconsistent with the needs of patients, thus then, the nurses who should provide broad services for patients can only address limited treatment tasks that are ordered by the physicians, consequently, this results in ethical problems. They also suffer from physical illness, mental disorder, and emotional exhaustion [7–15].

Moreover, nurses might encounter numerous ambiguous beliefs that might affect provision of quality of care [16–19]. Scarcity of medical equipment and complex clinical problems in the therapeutic system has directed an increment in the ethical difficulties encountered by nurses. In addition, sometimes ethical issues arise when procedures are performed without informed consent from the patient, during this time nurses will be exposed to internal as well as external controls to reply to the desires of patients [20, 21].

Furthermore, advance in technology, greater improvement in management and intervention, reduced hospitalization capacity, and an increase of awareness in patients about their rights have led to focus on an improved ethical climate [22]. Organizational citizenship manners are both social and psychological activity, which is favorable to sustaining and improving the quality of care [23–25].

Nursing activities are associated with organizational work climate in various angles. Within the hospital setting, the nurses' activities are documented as an integral component in the provision of quality health care and it is very important in terms of individual choices, such as promotion and retention [26]. Performance is the process of assessing how well employees accomplish their tasks as per a set of standards and providing that evidence to responsible bodies, and nurses' performance is defined as how well the task is performed in line with a set norm. It denotes the forthcoming possibility to carry out certain actions in order to fruitfully attain set goals within the given time frame and constraints of the stakeholders [27–29]. Structural citizenship manners comprise a group of professional conducts, which are not a portion of the character's proper responsibilities. It is done by the employees lacking the formal development system of the institute. Yet, it points to effective and improved fulfillment of organizational roles and responsibilities [30].

Moral philosophy with core values is very vital for nurses while they provide services, including the consideration of the patient's wants, needs, and preferences. Therefore, nursing has been considered to be an ethical-laden practice [31, 32]. Moral sensitivity is the ability to become aware of patients' vulnerability and recognize ethical conflicts. Thus, it is considered the first step in ethical decision-making [33–38]. The aim of this chapter is to provide information on hospital ethical climate and its influence on clinical nurses' perception on their organizational citizenship performance. This chapter recognized the ethical climate and job satisfaction among clinical nurses and dimensions of job design.

2. Ethical climate and job satisfaction among clinical nurses

According to the studies conducted in different countries, job satisfaction is a complex and multidimensional thought which denotes an internal state of mind of an individual. The level of job happiness is determined by the difference between what a person adds to his or her job and what he or she anticipates [39, 40]. The finding of different studies showed that ethical standards in an organization encourage esteem among the staff members and make them more motived and committed to their performance, which results in job satisfaction and organizational success. In addition, it produces a sense of possession and diminishes loneliness in employees, which increases the accomplishment of the organization [20, 41–47].

The study results showed that job satisfaction of employees leads to several positive behavioral outcomes at work. Like, it brings about productive work behavior, enables employees to satisfy customers/patients, and creates customer experience at work. Furthermore, the concept of satisfaction for healthcare employees has been described as a positive feeling of contentment that individuals obtain from their job while working for a corporate organization. The importance of job satisfaction of nurses on patients' provision of care, patient satisfaction, patient result, and overall healthcare provision cannot be over-underlined, as employee's job satisfaction is critical in the day-to-day lifecycle of the employees. It has been well-known that low job satisfaction is the chief source of employee turnover among healthcare service workers [48, 49]. Proposed that job satisfaction is an employee's feeling about his or her work environment, which includes the job itself, supervisor, workgroup, organization, and life [50, 51].

On the other hand, poor job satisfaction and improper ethical climate are factors that promote understaffed wards, loss of motivation, and increase nurses' turnover [41, 52, 53]. A study conducted in Ethiopia showed that more than half of nurses responded that they were not satisfied with their jobs [54]. According to the study done in Iran, the result revealed that nurses' perception of ethical climate and job satisfaction in hospital was at a moderate level [41].

The study finding showed that improved nurses' perception of the hospital's ethical climates could enhance their organizational citizenship behavior and at the same time it has a critical role in promoting job satisfaction and organizational commitment of nurses [42, 55]. Provided that place of work concerns remains to be seen as a major cause of the healthcare shortage it is clear that a positive ethical climate is a significant element of nurses' job satisfaction [56].

The satisfaction of healthcare workers is seriously affected, especially in developing countries, which is the major justification for turnover intention to foreign countries where they will be appreciated and provided with better working conditions [57].

Studies results revealed that the association between the work environment and job satisfaction across varied background grounds. The idea of the work environment and job satisfaction is to grow with time owing to its impact on the larger society [58–61]. The main factors that affect job satisfaction and nurses' assessments of the quality of care provided at the case team level are the practice environment and the availability of adequate resources [22, 62, 63].

Positive climate in hospitals may decline moods of being alone and it has a positive impact on output and patient satisfaction. A positive ethical climate improves job satisfaction, decreasing turnover, and nursing shortages [64, 65]. Satisfied nurses tend to be more fruitful and dedicated to their employers, and a direct correlation has been shown between staff satisfaction and patient satisfaction in health-care organizations [66, 67].

Self-worth has been recognized as a defensive factor alongside psychological suffering among nurses, and is positively correlated with nurses' well-being and is related to job satisfaction through both direct and indirect effects [9–12].

3. Dimensions of job design

Hackman and Oldham, suggest five dimensions of job design that influence on psychology mechanisms that profit employees and job results. It takes into consideration employees different sights as curbing factors of association between job features and job outcome factors [67]. In this regard, they established the five job characteristics as follows:

3.1 Skill variety

This explains the extent to which a job demands various skills, ability and capacity from an individual employee in achieving a set task. This is said to drive employee satisfaction when an employee has the necessary skills to perform a certain task and opportunity for training where there is a deficiency of required skills.

3.2 Task identity

It describes the aspect in which job demands realizing complete and identifying the part of the job task that will help in accomplishing the work from beginning to the end with a visible, marked, and positive outcome. This also is said to motivate employees and gear them to be happy on the job.

3.3 Task significance

This emphasizes the extent to which a job has a cogent influence on the well-being of other employees, or how it affects other employees, within and outside the firm.

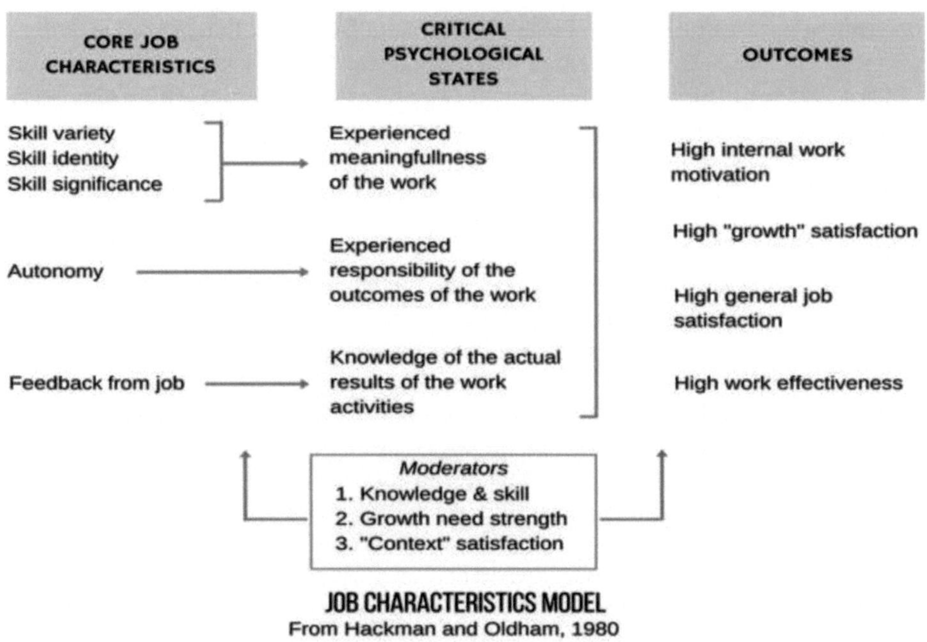

Source: Hackman and Oldman, (1980, p. 90)

Figure 1.
Job characteristics model.

In other words, employees' understanding of several other individuals who depend on the work they are performing is a crucial point in their satisfaction.

3.4 Job autonomy

This describes the degree of independent judgment to make informed decisions and discretion regarding the assigned task given to individual employees. In other words, the liberty to expand on the job and responsibilities is given to the employees to perform their duties and functions effectively. Autonomy in the workplace provides employees with a sense of job ownership and makes them feel in charge of the work, which largely steers up the satisfaction in an individual employee.

3.5 Job feedback

It explains a process by which reporting managers, superiors, and peers at work offer constructive suggestions to employees on the assigned task, which allows improvement and possible enhanced productive work behavior. According to the theorist, this stimulates the dedication of employees and makes them happy on the job (**Figure 1**).

4. Conclusion

As the major motor in the change of health-care system, nurses have more interaction time with patients in day-to-day clinical activities.

Hospital ethical climates have become a crucial working area element for nurses to prepare and apply ethical judgments.

Health-care professionals have a cluster of principles and attitudes that consist of acknowledgments, feelings, and actions, which are a reflection of one's professional values.

Effective nurses' nature is a positive professional attitude and professional values.

Job satisfaction is indispensable in the daily life of the workforce, and the mechanism that drives job satisfaction requires the attention of the management of corporate organizations.

Author details

Teketel Ermias Geltore
Midwifery Department, School of Nursing and Midwifery, College of Health Sciences and Medicine, Wachemo University, Durame, Ethiopia

*Address all correspondence to: teketelermias@gmail.com

References

[1] Al Hamdan Z, Bani Issa H. The role of organizational support and self-efficacy on work engagement among registered nurses in Jordan: A descriptive study. Journal of Nursing Management. 2021;**12**:1-11. DOI: 10.1111/JONM.13456

[2] Zangeneh A., Lebni JY, Azar FEF, Sharma M, Kianipour N, Azizi SA, et al. A study of the communication skills in health care and the role of demographic variables (a case study of the nurses at the education). 2019

[3] Esmaelzadeh F, Abbaszadeh A, Borhani F, Peyrovi H. Ethical sensitivity in nursing ethical leadership: A content analysis of Iranian nurses experiences. Open Nursing Journal. 2017;**11**:1-13

[4] Martin D, Cullen B. Continuities and extensions of ethical climate theory: A meta-analytic review. Journal of Business Ethics. 2006;**69**(2):175-194

[5] Choi S, Cheung K, Pang S. Attributes of nursing work environment as predictors of registered nurses' job satisfaction and intention to leave. Journal of Nursing Management. 2012;**21**:1-11

[6] Aiswarya B, Ramasundaram G. A Study on Interference of Work–Life Conflict between Organizational Climate and Job Satisfaction of Women Employees in the Information Technology Sector. Asia-Pacific Journal of Management Research and Innovation. 2012;**8**:351-360

[7] Mousazadeh S, Yektatalab S, Momennasab M, Parvizy S. Job satisfaction and related factors among Iranian intensive care unit nurses. BMC Research Notes. 2018;**11**(1):1-5

[8] Kunaviktikul W, Wichaikhum O, Nantsupawat A, Nantsupawat R, Chontawan R, Klunklin A, et al. Nurses' extended work hours: Patient, nurse and organizational outcomes. International Nursing Review. 2015;**62**(3):386-393

[9] Ndejjo R, Musinguzi G, Yu X, Buregyeya E, Musoke D, Wang JS, et al. Occupational health hazards among healthcare workers in Kampala, Uganda. Journal of Environmental Public Health. 2015;**2015**:913

[10] Azizoğlu F, Köse A, Gül H. Self-reported environmental health risks of nurses working in hospital surgical units. International Nursing Review. 2019;**66**(1):87-93

[11] Jamali J, Roustaei N, Ayatollahi SM, Sadeghi E. Factors affecting minor psychiatric disorder in Southern Iranian Nurses: A latent class regression analysis. Nursing Midwifery Studies. 2015;**4**(2):e28017

[12] Cheung T, Yip P. Depression, anxiety and symptoms of stress among Hong Kong nurses: A cross-sectional study. International Journal of Environmental Research and Public Health. 2015;**12**(9):11072-11100

[13] Cummings J. Compassion in Practice: Nursing, Midwifery & Care Staff – Our Vision & Strategy. London: NHS Commissioning Board; 2012

[14] Mousazadeh S, Yektatalab S, Momennasab M, Parvizy S. Impediments to the formation of intensive care nurses' professional identify. Nursing Ethics. 2019;**26**(6):1873-1885

[15] Yektatalab S, Momennasab M, Parvizy S, Mousazadeh N. Improving nurses' job satisfaction: An action research study. Systemic Practice and Action Research. 2021;**2021**:1-18

[16] Belle M-J. Critical Care Nurses' Professional Identity Constructions in an Australian Intensive Care Unit: Contextual and Contingent. University of Tasmania, Human Research Ethical Committee; 2017

[17] Mahdaviseresht R, Atashzadeh-Shoorideh F, Borhani F. Correlation between moral sensitivity and moral courage in nurses of selected hospitals affiliated to Tabriz University of Medical Sciences in 2014. Iranian Journal of Medical Ethics and History of Medicine. 2015;**8**(3):27-39

[18] Ulrich C, Taylor C, Soeken K, et al. Everyday ethics: Ethical issues and stress in nursing practice. Other. 2010;**66**:1-15

[19] Jafree SR, Zakar R, Fischer F, Zakar MZ. Ethical violations in the clinical setting: The hidden curriculum learning experience of Pakistani nurses. BMC Medical Ethics. 2015;**16**:16

[20] Suhonen R, Stolt M, Virtanen H, Leino-Kilpi H. Organizational ethics: A literature review. Nursing Ethics. 2011;**18**(3):285-303

[21] Organ DW. Organizational citizenship behavior: It's construct clean-up time. Human Performance. 1997;**10**:85-97

[22] Cerit B, Özveren H. Effect of hospital ethical climate on the nurses' moral sensitivity. The European Research Journal. 2019;**5**(2):282-290

[23] Talachi RK, Gorji MB, Boerhannoeddin AB. An investigation of the role of job satisfaction in employees' organizational citizenship behavior. Collegium Antropologicum. 2014;**38**:429-436

[24] Dzeng E, Curtis JR. Understanding Ethical Climate, Moral Distress, and Burnout: A Novel Tool and a Conceptual Framework. BMJ Quality and Safety. Oct 2018;**27**(10):766-770. DOI: 10.1136/bmjqs-2018-007905

[25] Luo Z, Shi K, Li W, Mia D. Construct of job performance: Evidence from Chinese's Military Soldiers. Asian Journal of Psychology. 2008;**11**:222-223

[26] Nabirye R. Occupational Stress, Job Satisfaction and Job Performance among Hospital Nurses in Kampala Uganda. Makerere University; 2011

[27] Yu M, Hamid S, Ijab M, Soo H. The balanced score card (E-BSC) for measuring academic staff performance excellence. High Education. 2009;**57**:813-828

[28] Mathis RL, Jackson JH. Human Resource Management. 9th ed. Cincinnati, Ohio: South Western College Publishing; 2000

[29] Makaroff KS, Storch J, Pauly B, Newton L. Searching for ethical leadership in nursing. Nursing Ethics. 2014;**21**:642-658

[30] Lützén K, Dahlqvist V, Eriksson S, Norberg A. Developing the concept of moral sensitivity in health care practice. Nursing Ethics. 2006;**13**(2):187-196

[31] Laine C, Davidoff F. Patient-centered medicine: A professional evolution. Journal of the American Medical Association. 1996;**275**(2):152-156

[32] Han SS, Kim J, Kim YS, Ahn S. Validation of a Korean version of the moral sensitivity questionnaire. Nursing Ethics. 2010;**17**(1):99-105

[33] Lützén K, Cronqvist A, Magnusson A, Andersson L. Moral stress: Synthesis of a concept. Nursing Ethics. 2003;**10**(3):312-322

[34] DeKeyser GF, Berkovitz K. Surgical nurses' perceptions of ethical dilemmas, moral distress and quality of care. Journal of Advanced Nursing. 2012;**68**(7):1516-1525

[35] Kim S. Development and initial psychometric evaluation of nurses' ethical decision making around end-of-life-care scale in Korea. Journal of Hospice and Palliative Nursing. 2011;**13**(2):97-105

[36] Krautscheid LC. Defining professional nursing accountability: A literature review. Journal of Professional Nursing. 2014;**30**(1):43-47

[37] Lützén K, Evertzon M, Nordin C. Moral sensitivity in psychiatric practice. Nursing Ethics. 1997;**4**(6):472-482

[38] Farsi Z, Dehghan-Nayeri N, Negarandeh R, Broomand S. Nursing profession in Iran: An overview of opportunities and challenges. Japan Journal of Nursing Science. 2010;**7**(1):9-18

[39] Zarea K, Negarandeh R, Dehghan-NayeriI N, Rezaei-Adaryani M. Nursing staff shortages and job satisfaction in Iran. Nursing & Health Sciences. 2009;**11**(3):326-331

[40] Malloy D, Hadjistavropoulos T, Mccarthy E, et al. Culture, organisational climate and ontology: An international study of nurses. Nursing Ethics. 2009;**16**(6):719-733. DOI: 10.1177/0969733009342636

[41] Huang C, You C, Tsai M. A multidimensional analysis of ethical climate, job satisfaction, organizational commitment, and organizational citizenship behaviors. Nursing Ethics. 2012;**19**:513-529

[42] Abou Hashish EA. Relationship between ethical work climate and nurses' perception of organizational support, commitment, job satisfaction and turnover intent. Nursing Ethics. 2017;**24**:151-166

[43] Feather J, Mcgillis Hall L, Trbovich P, Baker GR. An integrative review of nurses' prosaically behaviors contributing to work environment optimization, organizational performance and quality of care. Journal of Nursing Management. 2018;**26**:769-781

[44] Özlük B, Baykal Ü. Organizational citizenship behavior among nurses: The influence of organizational trust and job satisfaction. Florence Nightingale Journal of Nursing. 2020;**28**:333-340

[45] Eroğluer K, Ö. Y. The effect of ethical leadership behavior on perceived organizational climate: Mediating role of work loneliness. Journal of Business Res-Turk. 2015;7:280-308

[46] Süreci Y. Hospital workers' perception of ethical climate. The Journal of Academic Social Science Studies. 2015;**35**:425-437

[47] Chamal GS, Dilina H. Employee satisfaction and related factors among public health workers in Sri-Lanka: A case study on regional directorate of hambanthota. JOJ Nurse Health Care. 2018;**8**(4):1-7

[48] Ezeja EB, Azodo CC, Ehizele AO, Ehigiator O, Oboro HO. Assessment of job satisfaction and working conditions of Nigerian oral health workers. International Journal of Biomedical and Health Sciences. 2010;**6**(3):143-150

[49] Castle NG, Engberg J, Anderson RA. Job satisfaction of nursing home administrators and turnover. Medical Care Research and Review. 2007;**64**:191-211

[50] Porter LW, Lawer RE. Organizational, work, and personal factors in employee turnover and absenteeism. Psychological Bulletin. 1973;**88**:151-176

[51] Asegid A, Belachew T, Yimam E. Factors influencing job satisfaction and anticipated turnover among nurses in

Sidama zone public health facilities. Nursing Research & Practice. 2014;**2014**:26

[52] Afsar B, Shahjehan A, Cheema S, Javed F. The effect of perceiving a calling on Pakistani nurses' organizational commitment, organizational citizenship behavior, and job stress. Journal of Transcultural Nursing. 2018;**29**:540-547

[53] Government of Ethiopia and the World Bank. Health Sector Review, Ethiopian Social Sector Studies. 1st ed. Addis Ababa: Mega; 2004

[54] Taraz Z, Loghmani L, Abbaszadeh A, Ahmadi F, Safavibiat Z, Borhani F. The relationship between ethical climate of hospital and moral courage of nursing staff. Electronic Journal of Genetic Medicine. 2019;**16**(2):1-6

[55] American Association of Colleges of Nursing. The essentials of baccalaureate education for professional nursing practice. The American Association of Colleges of Nursing; 2002. (Retrieved from http://www.aacn.nche.edu/education-resources/BaccEssentials08.pdf)

[56] Kovnet CT, Brewer CS, Fatehi F, Jun J. What does the nurse turnover rate mean and what is the rate? Policy Politics and Nursing Practice. 2014;**15**(3/4):64-71

[57] Aiken LH, Sloane DM, Bruyneel L, Van den Heede K, Sermeus W. Consortium nurses' reports of working conditions and hospital quality of care in 12 countries in Europe. International Journal of Nursing Studies. 2013;**50**(2):143-153

[58] Chaudhury S. Job satisfaction of hospital staff: An emerging challenge. Medical Journal of Dr. D.Y. Patil University. 2015;**8**(2):129-138

[59] Khunou SH, Davhana-Maselesele M. Level of job satisfaction amongst nurses in the north-west province, South-Africa. Post-occupation specific dispensation. Curationis. 2016;**39**(1):1

[60] Kim JM. The difference in life satisfaction and job satisfaction of nursing teachers depending on their socio-demographic characteristics. Advanced Science and Technology Letters. 2015;**103**:197-201

[61] Impacts of unit-level nurse practice environment and burnout on nurse-reported outcomes: A multilevel modeling approach. Journal of Clinical Nursing. 2010;**19**:1664-1674

[62] Hinno S, Partanen P, Vehviläinen-Julkunen K. Hospital nurses' work environment, quality of care provided and career plans. Journal of Nursing Review. 2011;**58**:255-262

[63] Aiken LH, Sloane DM, Clarke S, Poghosyan L, Cho E, You L, et al. Importance of work environments on hospital outcomes in nine countries. International Journal for Quality in Health Care. 2011;**23**:357-364

[64] Rivaz M, Rakhshan M, Vizeshfar F, Setoodegan E. Validation of the Iranian Version of the Hospital Ethical Climate Survey. Journal of Nursing Measurement. 2020;**28**(1):JNM-D-18-00086. DOI: 10.1891/JNM-D-18-00086

[65] Al-Almeri AS. Job satisfaction and organizational commitment for nurses. Saudi Medical Journal. 2000;**21**:531-535

[66] Tzeng HM. The influence of nurses' working motivation and job satisfaction on intention to quit: An empirical investigation in Taiwan. International Journal of Nursing Studies. 2002;**39**:867-878

[67] Hackman JR, Oldham GR. Work Redesign. Reading, MA: Addison-Wesley; 1980

Chapter 5

Therapeutic Effect of Barley on Cardiovascular Diseases

Madiha Khan Niazi, Zainab Saeed, Sahar Imran and Farooq Hassan

Abstract

Barley is a fantastic food option for those with various illnesses as well as for those who want to lead a healthy lifestyle. This cereal is a great source of soluble dietary fiber, particularly beta-glucans, and it also includes vital vitamins and minerals. For its excellent antioxidant activity and as a source of vitamins and minerals, green barley is advised. Depending on phytonutrients such as glucan, phenolics, flavonoid, lignans, tocols, sitosterol, and folic, regular consumption of whole wheat grain and its hydroethanolic extracts decreases the risk of chronic ailments (hyperglycemia, malignancy, overweight, cardiac disease, and so on). Barley and its products in recent years have gained an importance due to its counteractive components, which play potent role against cardiovascular diseases by lowering down the oxidative stress and improving high-density lipoprotein, further lowering down low-density lipoprotein, VLDL ratios further regulating insulin levels, and lowering down the spike in blood glucose levels showing potent antioxidative and cardiovascular functions. Due to their abundance in these nutrients, barley is effective in promoting healthy bodily function. To enjoy all of the advantages of barley, barley grain is a wonderful option.

Keywords: barley, medicinal, therapeutic, cardiovascular disease, herb

1. Introduction

Elevated blood pressure, coronary heart disease (CHD), heart failure, and stroke are all examples of cardiovascular disease (CVD), a condition that affects the heart and blood arteries. Elevated blood pressure, coronary heart disease (CHD), heart failure, and stroke are all examples of cardiovascular disease (CVD), a condition that affects the heart and blood arteries. This disease is usually related to fatty deposits, which are buildup inside arteries, and there is chance of blood clots. Strokes and heart attacks are acute events, which are mainly caused by obstruction of blood from going from the heart to brain. Heart muscles and valves are affected by the heart disease; this can also result in arrhythmias. Heart and blood vessel disorders that impact the anatomy and physiology of the circulatory system are referred to as cardiovascular diseases [1]. Hypertension, ischemic heart disease, peripheral vascular disease, stroke, rheumatic heart disease, heart failure, valvular heart disease, and a congenital cardiac condition are the most prevalent forms of CVD [2].

Blood clots or hemorrhages from a brain blood artery can both result in strokes. A total of 811,940 deaths in 2009 were attributable to CVD, making up 32.8% of all fatalities in the country. There are 82 million Americans who suffer from one or more types of CVD. The two types of CVD risk factors are modifiable and non-modifiable. Gender, age, ethnicity, genetics are all considered as non-modifiable factors. On the other hand, smoking, body weight, blood pressure, lipid, lipoprotein levels are all modifiable factors. CVD can be avoided or reduced by adopting health-promoting habits that target the modifiable risk factors. One can reduce their risk of acquiring CVD by engaging in exercise, eating a healthy diet, taking medicine, and quitting smoking [2].

Strong epidemiological data support the idea that CVD occurs more frequently in families. According to Framingham Study, researchers revealed that not less than one parent with CVD quadrupled a person's 8-year chance of developing the disease in men and raised it by 70% in women. The extra risk was unrelated to other risk variables such as age, body mass index (BMI), diabetes, total/high-density lipoprotein cholesterol (HDL-C) ratio, systolic blood pressure (SBP), antihypertensive therapy, and current smoking status. History of family is considered as medical and health details of members in family. First- and second-degree relatives' medical and health information is the most useful because it shares bout 50 and 25%, respectively, of our genes. The presence of common genes that may be responsible for polygenic (complex) illnesses, habitats, and gene-environment interactions that may affect risk are all reflected in family history, which acts as a connection between genetics and genomics in clinical practice. Family history (FH) is a stand-alone CVD risk factor that can be possibly used as a screening tool to detect CVD risk, particularly in asymptomatic young adults [2]. Increased plasma cholesterol has been shown to be a significant CVD risk factor. By boosting LDL expression and lowering LDL oxidation, tea and its polyphenols may lower plasma cholesterol levels. Tea may prevent the development of atherosclerosis by lowering antifibrinolysin, eliminating reactive oxygen species, and causing hypolipemia. In general, tea and its polyphenols may be useful nutritional components for the reduction of cancer and cardiovascular disease (CVD) [3].

1.1 Causes

Cardiovascular diseases (CVDs) are becoming more common over the world and are currently regarded as the main cause of death in both emerging and industrialized nations. The prevalence of these diseases has increased and reached alarming levels in recent decades as a result of the quick economic development and increasingly Westernized lifestyle. The well-known causes of CVDs include behavioral risk factors such as a harmful diet (high in fat, salt, and sugar), physical inactivity, injurious alcohol and tobacco use, a high BMI, a high waist-to-hip ratio, and metabolic risk factors such as hyperglycemia, hyperlipidemia, and high blood pressure. Inflammatory rheumatic disorders are linked to an increased risk of cardiovascular disease (CVD) [4]. High blood pressure, also known as hypertension, atherosclerosis or artery blockages, inactivity, obesity, sleep apnea, excessive alcohol consumption, stress, air pollution, chronic obstructive pulmonary disease, radiation therapy, smoking, poor sleep and hygiene, high blood cholesterol, also known as hyperlipidemia, diabetes, a high-fat, high-carbohydrate diet, or other conditions that reduce lung function are all risk factors for CVD [5]. The growth and progression of CVD are also mediated by metals such as lead, cadmium, and arsenic, which are among the top 10 environmental pollutants of concern according to the WHO [6]. Multiple comorbid illnesses are frequently present in cardiovascular disease (CVD) patients, which can complicate treatment decisions, lower mortality, and interact with one another. One of the most significant comorbidities of CVD is chronic obstructive pulmonary disease (COPD), which has considerable effects on individuals with ischemic heart disease, stroke, arrhythmia, and heart failure. Less physical activity is linked to COPD, which causes systemic inflammation and oxidative stress and shares risk factors with CVD such as smoking and age [7].

1.2 Signs and symptoms

It has been established that sleep apnea has a negative effect on health. Among its severe side effects are chest pain, breathlessness, feeling dizzy, faint, swollen limbs, fatigue, weakness, very fast or slow heartbeat, numbness in legs or arms, stress, physically inactive, being obese or overweight [8]. Heartburn, nausea, vomiting, pressure, or squeezing in the chest, pain radiating to the neck, shoulder, back, arm, or jaw, chest discomfort, clamminess, and cold sweats. Commonly in women symptoms, which are seen are as follows: Slight discomfort in the back, chest, arm, neck, or jaw, sudden onset of weakness, shortness of breath, weariness, and a feeling of systemic sickness (without chest pain) as shown in **Figure 1** [9].

The relative chance of developing hypercholesterolemia is more in men that in young women; in postmenopausal stage, lipid profile is adverse, with LDL and total cholesterol, which go high by 10–14%, respectively, without any change in high-density lipoproteins. Therefore, in women with a borderline premenopausal profile, postmenopausal reassessment of lipids is crucial to take into account. However, LDL

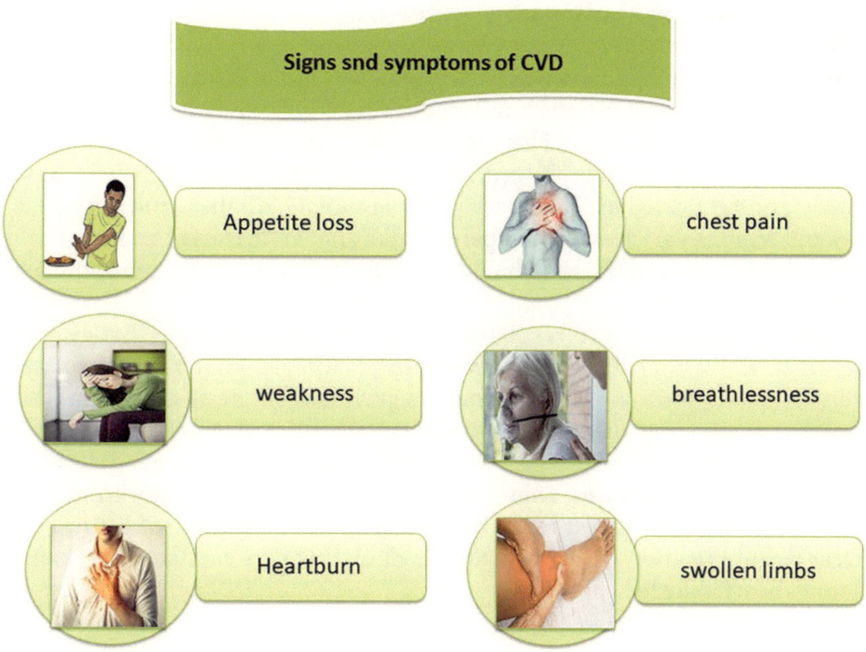

Figure 1.
Sign and symptoms of CVD.

lowering with statins lowers CHD mortality to a comparable degree as in males, even though mean LDL is higher in women over 65 than in males [10].

1.3 Prevalence

The annual rate of cardiovascular death has been calculated to be around 9%. The main cause of death worldwide is cardiovascular disease (CVD). According to estimates, 17.9 million deaths worldwide in 2019 were attributable to CVDs, or 32% of all fatalities. Heart attacks and strokes were to blame for 85% of these deaths. In low- and middle-income nations, almost 75% of CVD fatalities occur. In 2019, CVDs were responsible for 38% of the 17 million premature deaths (before the age of 70) caused by noncommunicable diseases.

By addressing behavioral risk factors such as tobacco use, unhealthy eating and obesity, inactivity, and problematic alcohol consumption, the majority of cardiovascular illnesses can be kept away. Initial diagnosis of cardiovascular disease is crucial in order to start treatment with counseling and medication. Australian population ranged between 1.0 and 2.0%, in Western countries (United Kingdom, Germany, and the United States), it is about 25% [11]. In Pakistan, it was found that genetic predisposition caused the disease in 72.9% of men and 79.9% of females, while 27.02% of males and 20.99% of females had CVD without any family history. In South Asia, ratio of heart disease is 24.2%, and in East Asia, it is 21.3% [12].

The prevalence of CVD was 14.8 (urban) and 9.7% (rural) among Delhi's urban and rural groups (rural). Overall, death rates are the highest for both men and women in Punjab, Eastern and Northeastern States, and South Indian States, while they are the lowest in Central Indian States [13].

2. Effect of barley on cardiovascular disease

Hordeum vulgare, often known as barley, is a plant in the Poaceae family. It is estimated that barley was initially cultivated from its native relative *Hordeum spontaneum* roughly 10,000 years ago. There is proof that the Fertile Crescent's Israel-Jordan region is where barley was initially grown [14] as well as it is been clarified that barley was further domesticated in Tibet. Barley is a perennial herb that comes in both springs and winters varieties. Winter perennials are sown in the fall and need a duration of cold weather until they will bloom. Modern cultivars also include both hulled and hulless variants [15].

One of the oldest cereal crops still being cultivated today is barley. Barley contains dietary fiber, which contributes to many health advantages. Phenolic acid, folate, vitamin E, lignans, phenolic acids, flavonoids, phytosterols are all present in whole grain barley. These phytochemicals have substantial antioxidant, cholesterol-lowering properties, and inhibition of cell growth that may be helpful in reducing the risk of developing specific diseases. Therefore, in barley there is high concentration of phytochemicals as shown in **Figure 2**. Barley products were permitted by the Food and Drug Administration (FDA) to make the claim that they cut down the chance of developing heart issue [4].

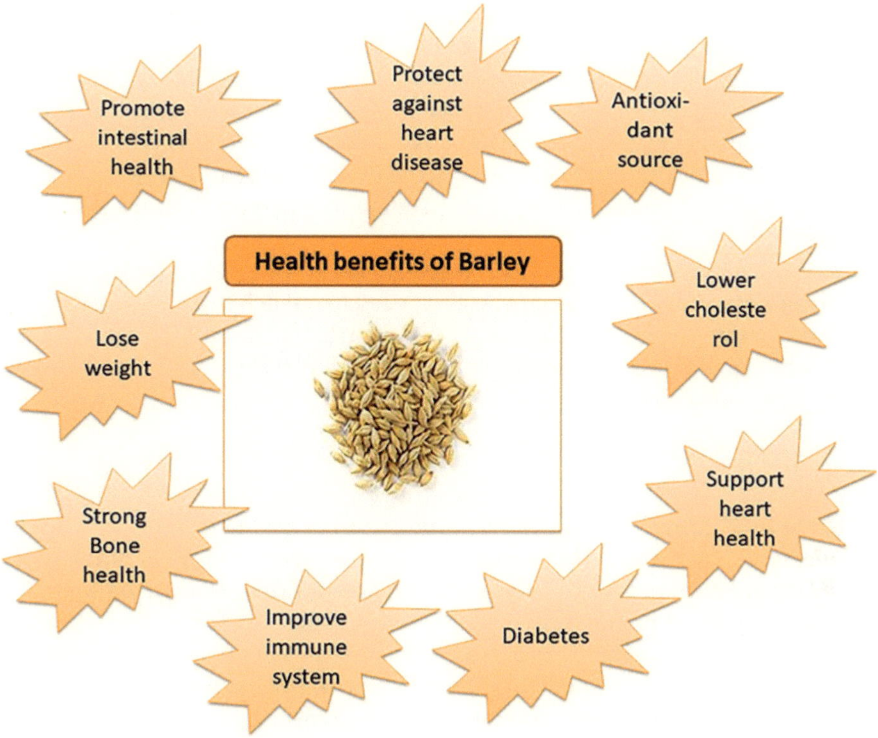

Figure 2
Health benefits of barley.

3. Potential barley-based health products

3.1 Multigrain atta

The amount of soluble and insoluble fiber in wheat atta is increased with the help of hulled barley (flour). This could lower the glycemic load of flatbreads, a dietary staple, which is consumed particularly in northern India [16].

3.2 Multigrain biscuits and bread

The addition of hulless barley may enhance the bread's and the biscuits' nutritional benefits. Experimental investigations at ICAR-IIWBR have demonstrated the viability of barley-based biscuits. Similar to that, barley malts could be used to flavor cookies.

3.3 Barley flakes

Breakfast cereals such as flakes can be made from hulled barley; however, flavoring is required to make the cereals more palatable [16].

3.4 Ready-to-eat and drink sattu: traditionally beverage called as sattu is made from barley or gram flour

The Hadiths admonish sattu (finely ground barley) being a nutritional food. Yet another health item named as Talbina is made by mixing milk and honey with the dried barley powder and by adding Sattoo in it. This meal is very beneficial for the sick and the bereaved, and it also provides the patient's heart a rest and stimulates it.

In accordance with Ibn al-Qayyim, barley-enriched water when boiled to that extent that only it reduces to three quarters is used to quench thirst and leads in treating skin lesions. Hagiwara investigated that barley is enriched with high sodium content, which maintains calcium levels in the blood, further aids in dissolving the deposits of calcium in joints.

3.4.1 Production

In the year of 2016/2017, worldwide production of barley was 145 million metric tons. Due to massive production annually, barley is placed in fourth number after rice, wheat, and corn produce. Mainly those countries that produce barley in massive amount are Russia, Germany, France, Ukraine, Australia, and Canada. An easily grown, widely accepted, and robust crop, it has now been grown in more than 100 countries worldwide. Primarily, it is grown over in warm countries but its varied growth can also be seen in some tropics regions. About 60% of barley crop is utilized for animal feeding purposes, and the remaining percentage is utilized for majorly for brewing purposes. Previously to till today, barley production has seen an increase of about 60% among European countries. This is partly attributable to the development of more productive cultivars with improved disease and pest resistance. Meanwhile, significant improvement in agricultural practices also posed a major development [17].

4. Types

4.1 Barley grass

The grass of barley is regarded as more than just the best nutraceutical having effective properties required for the cell nourishment with detoxifying effects in humans. Barley grass also contains potent functionalized substances, which have a variety of health-promoting properties [5]. It has ability to oppose more than 20 chronic inflammations or ailments, which is due to the presence of gamma aminobutyric acid, flavonols, SODs, potassium-calcium, vitamin, and tryptophan's modulatory actions in its grass [18]. The World Health Organization daily consumption targets of less salt's intake (less than 2 g) and improved K consumption (more than 3.5 g) can be achieved with barley grass powder. Barley increased the sterols deposition with the help of LTP2 gene modulation that plays potent effect in environmental stressed reactions of moderating intracellular lipidases transportation [19].

4.2 Barley grains

Among cereal crops, they offer the high practicable index (less glycemic index, higher glucans, and starches), as well as the best antioxidant capabilities. A class of polysaccharides known as soluble fiber glucans can be present in seaweed, barley, oats, morels, and *Saccharomyces cerevisiae* [20]. Whole barley flour should be consumed regularly on a daily basis to prevent chronic diseases, particularly diabetes, colonic cancer, hypercholesterolemia, hypertension, and gall-bladder stones [21]. Despite the fact that barley grains have contributed significantly to human health outcomes, there are many major ways through which barley can benefit human health by their modulatory mechanisms [21].

5. Chemical composition

Barley is not just a significant feeder, malts, and food crops in several countries throughout the world, as well as the greatest cereal resource of functional component among the most widespread variety of multifunctional cereal crops and is incredibly full of beneficial nutrients. Particularly fiber, phenols, flavones, phytosterol, alkylresorcinols, benzoxazinoids, lignans, tocols, and folic acid, which have antidiabetes, anticancer, antiobesity, preventive cardiovascular disease, antioxidant, antiproliferative, and cholesterol lowering properties. Whole barley grains and its outermost grain layers are densely packed with the beneficial nutrients [22], as beta-glucans (2.41~7.42%) and total tocols (40.9~81.6 μg/g) A lot more there are 64 compounds, out of which 27 among them are anthocyanides, 9 are flavanols, 9 are flavones glycosidase, and 19 are phenolic acids and aldehydones [23]. Among them, green malt is enriched with potent functional components, which showed (79.80%) of antioxidant potential, total phenol content (123.43 mg/100 g), (+)-catechin (70.06 mg/100 g), quercetin (31.78 mg/100 g), 1,2-dihydroxybenzene (38.21 mg/100 g), isorhamnetin (23.44 mg/100 g), and carotenoid (0.181 mg/100 g) [24]. The largest quantity of folate is found in the germ and outermost layers of hulled barley grains (103.3 mg/100 g). Maximum concentrate of calcium is recorded as 12, potassium is above 6, and iron is above 4 in the barley grains [25].

5.1 B-Glucan

The most prominent class of polysaccharides, which is found in barley, is B-glucan. In hulless wheat grain, -d-glucan has a molar mass of 571.4 kDa and is composed of glucopyranosyl residues (1, 4, and 3), particularly its trisaccharide and tetrasaccharide, which account for 66.6% of the total cellulose subunits. To lower triglyceride levels and hence prevent diabetic condition, high blood pressure, cardiovascular diseases, and metabolic syndromes, B-glucans interact with the synthesis of bile salts and triglycerides in the stomach [26].

5.2 Polyphenols and flavonoids in hull barley

Anti-inflammatory, anticancer, and antioxidative potentials depend on the phenolic acid compound concentration [27]. Most abundantly available phenols in barley are 4-hydroxybenzoic acid (17.6%), isomers of hydroxycinnamic acid (15.2%), and ferulic acids (54.4%). Natural polyphenolic compounds, which are present in largest proportion, are the flavonoids. Class of anthocyanidins is majorly potent for human health related to flavonoids [28].

5.3 Phytosterols

In plants, structure of phytosterol showed similarity with cholesterol. Increased concentration of phytosterolic compounds is present in the outermost layer of grains of barley and ranges between 81.0 mg/100 g and 114.3 mg/100 g, among which β-sitosterol is 46:6 ± 0:1 mg/100 g and campesterol is 17:1 ± 0:2 mg/100 g. Other potent phytosterolic compound concentration includes stigma sterol (3.9 mg/100 g), brassicasterol, δ5-avenasterol, stigmastanol, stigmastadienol, and other minor sterols (δ5- and δ7-avenasterols, δ7-stigmastenol, and stigmastadienol: 8:6 ± 0:1 mg/100 g) [26–28].

5.4 Tocols

Most prominently fat-soluble antioxidative compound for human health is vitamin E containing eight stereoisomers. Spring barley compounds have increased alpha-tocopherol concentration among its other classes. Alpha-tocopherol concentration in barley is about 0.860–3.15 mg/100 g dry weight. Tocochromanol concentration in barley is 50% in pericarp, >37% in endo-sperm, which is less than 13% in germ layer; around 85% tocotrienols and fat-soluble phenolic compounds in germ layer (80%) were significant than that which is found in peri-carp (20%) [29].

6. Functioning ingredients in barley grass and barley grain against chronic illnesses

β-Glucans can be used as candidates for the medication in the treatment of human chronic diseases (**Table 1**).

6.1 Mechanism of action

Gamma amino butyric acid ($C_4H_9NO_2$) in barley grass improves sleeping disorders, lowers down high blood glucose levels, maintains hypertension, improves immune system function, has a protective role against liver, has a protective effect against depressant, regulates GIT tract function, potent inflammatory effect, shows oxidative effect, lowers down the risk of CVDs and heart, lessens down the risk of atopic dermatitis, and improves cognitive action. Gamma amino butyric acid and signaling pathways of dopamine are associated with sleep regulation [40]. GABA contains very potent intra-islet transient neurotransmitter, which maintains and regulates cell secretory effect from islets and shows potent inflammatory, immune regulator functional capabilities, which prevent diabetic condition and promote regenerative functional capabilities against beta-cell apoptotic lysis. GABA b receptor agonist baclofen ($C_{10}H_{12}ClNO_2$) affects toll-like receptor 3 and toll-like receptor 4 activity in glial and immunity boosting cells, which plays the key functional capabilities in neuronal-inflammatory ailments of the body [41].

Preventative action against chronic illnesses	Functioning component in grass	Functioning components in grains	References
Anti-hyperglycemic effect	Saponin; fiber calcium; AMPK, polyaminases; gamma alpha amino butyric acid, sodium oxide dismutase.	Beta-glucan; phenols polysaccharidases; tocolic compounds; phytosterolic compounds, resistant starches.	[30]
Lipid lowering effects or anti-obesity	Saponin; α-tocopherols; 2″-O- homovitexin, polysaccharidases	Polysaccharidases, starches, tocolic compounds, dietary fibers, polyphenolic compounds, polysaccharidases, phytosterolic compounds.	[31]
Anti-cancerous	Alkaline, flavonoids, chlorophyll; tricin; sodium oxide dismutase	Beta-glucan, phenolic compounds, arabinoxylanes, phytosterolic compounds, lignanes, resistant starches	[32, 33]
Anti-oxidative effects	Chlorophyll; lutonarin, saponarin; isoorientin, orientin; γ-tocopherol, glutathione; sodium oxide dismutase, flavonoid, (GABA)	Polyphenolics, anthocyanides, tocotrienols, polysaccharidases, (GABA)	[34, 35]
Immunomodulatory effects	Arabinoxylan; polysaccharide, gamma amino butyric acid	Beta-glucans, arabinoxylans	[36, 37]
Cardioprotective effects	potassium, Gamma amino butyric acid	Beta-D-Glucan	[38]
Blood pressure regulatory effect	Saponarin; lutonarin, potassium, calcium; gamma amino butyric acid	Beta-glucans	[39]
Bowel health regulatory effect	Soluble and insoluble fiber	Beta-glucans, soluble and insoluble fiber	[23]
Anti-preventative effect against CVD	Saponin; tryptophans, vitamins (retinol, thymine, tocopherol), sodium oxide dismutase; potassium, calcium; gamma amino butyric acid	Beta-glucans, arabinoxylans, polyphenolic compounds, phytosterolic compounds, lignanes, tocolic compounds, folic acid	[37–39]

Table 1.
Functioning ingredients in barley grass and barley grain against chronic illnesses.

Gamma amino butyric acid has the ability to prevent and cure CVDs, which are linked with platelet GP VI in such as hemorrhage and heart attack; majorly GABA retards activation of platelet, which is upregulated by convulsion, and increases clotting time of blood and the occlusioning times of platelets plugged forming [41].

7. Barley align with dietary guidelines for people with cardiovascular diseases

Barley, which is been considered as low-fat, fiber-enriched, whole-grain foodstuff in accordance with the nutrition recommendation used for the treatment of CVD regulated by the leading health promotion administration:

- The *Heart and Stroke Foundation of Canada* countersign intaking of food in relation with Food Guide by Canada's [42], which recommended that consume at least half of grains in the form of whole grains, eat a diversity of whole grains, and choose those whole grains items that are low fat, low sugar, or low salt [42].

- The *American Heart Association* countersign: consume those foods that are higher in whole grains, and half of grains consumption should come from whole grains. Whole grains are prescribed because it is the part of American Heart Association's lifestyle management regulations for lowering of both low-density lipoprotein cholesterol and hypertension [43].

- The Academic Curriculum of Nutrio-Dietetics—outlined on the health imputation of fiber—suggesting that, in accordance with CVD, consumption of dietary fiber from whole foods reduces blood pressure, regulates plasma lipids concentration, further reducing markers of inflammation [43].

8. Healthy effects of functional ingredients in barley grains against cardiovascular diseases

Barley beta-glucan has the ability to lower down low-density lipoprotein and highly dense lipoprotein cholesterol alongside retarding gut microbiotas leading to the prevention of cardiovascular diseases. Nutraceutical functions of the barley have been linked with cardio-protection health, which include polyphenols, phytosterol, lignin, tocolic acid, and folic acid [21]. Barley grains showed potent modulatory effect that only after 11–16 hours of their intake, and they maintained blood glucose levels and appetite hormones by their regulatory actions. Their mechanisms include GIT fermentation of indigestible carbohydrates [38]. Studies showed that the barley sprouted extricate, which contains 19.65 mg/g of overall polyphenolic concentration, and lowers down the extracellular cholesterol concentrations in mice to the levels of 24 and 18%, sequentially. Lignans, which are also found in barley, showed potent antioxidative functions when compared with vitamin E functionality, which is linked in lowering the risk factors of CVD [32].

Barley (1–3) Beta-d-glucan maintains and regulates cardio-protective ischemic effect showing 109% rates of survival chance after 30 minutes of having ischemic heart attack, reperfusion injury, lessens down the results of increase in the capillary at the amount of 12% and arterial density of about 18%, further expressing VEGF (88.7%) of hearts in rats [37].

Barley beta-d-glucan naturally activates the expression of manganese superoxide dismutase expression, which is maintained by anti-inflammation, metabolically and stressed-activated transcriptional factors, which are commonly expressed in relation to a commonly stressed condition, leading to the prevention of heart failure.

Beta-glucan lowers down coronary artery disease progression, hyperglycemia, and associated heart problems [38].

Tong et al. in the year 2015 proposed that diet-related beta-glucan found in hulled barley lowers down the plasma low-density lipo-protein cholestrolemic condition by initiating the evacuation of fecal triglycerides and maintaining the functioning of 3-OH-3-glutaryl-coenzyme A and cholesteric 7-α-hydroxylase in rats having hypercholesterolemic condition. Barley-enriched bran of 5–10% when added into the diet of these hypercholesterolemic rats improved the levels of lipases, lactate dehydrogenases, enzymes of liver, and creatinine kinases MB [39].

Wang et al. in the year 2016 conducted an analysis to find out the efficacy of B-glucan on cardiovascular ailments and to investigate that the altered composition of microbes is associated with biological activities of beta-glucan for improvement of the risk factors of cardiovascular diseases in mild hypercholesterolemia participants. Individuals received 3°g of increased molar mass (HMW), 3°g of lower molar mass (LMW), 5°g of low-molecular-weight barley β-glucan or wheat and rice for the time extension of 28 days. Results showed that intake of 3 g/day of high-molecular-weight Beta-glucan increases Bacteroidetes, which results in increased production of Prevotella when compared with 5°g low-molecular-weight Beta-glucan and 3°g low-molecular-weight Beta-Glucan, further suggesting that consuming higher-molar-mass β-glucan restricts the gut microbiota profiling, which is further linked with lower levels of risk-associated cardiovascular diseases markers [15].

Bachetti et al. in the year 2015 conducted an analysis, directed to investigate the nutraceuticals and functional possessions of barley-complemented vegetable-based soup and its protective effect against cardiovascular diseases. A total number of 38 participants took part, whose edibles were complemented for around 14°days including 250°g (Daily portion) of ready-to-eat soup being enriched with carotenes mainly (Beta-carotene and lutein), and its outcome was studied on its lipid profile and lipid peroxidation. After 14°days of treatment, blood serum concentrations of carotenes (lutein and Vitamin A precursor) and levels of overall plasma antioxidative capacities were increased. In addition to detection of reduction in lipid levels (total cholesterol and LDL-cholesterol), reduction in triglycerides oxidized markers (oxidized LDL low-density lipoprotein and lipid hydro peroxides) was seen in plasma levels of all the participants. As in terms of glycemic content of barley, it is of low glycmeic nature and does not blunt higher sugar levels. This study concluded that barley-enriched vegetable soup not only lowers down blood sugar level but also improves cardiovascular functions and serves as cardio-protection, further improving plasma lipid levels [44].

Xia et al. in the year 2018 hypothesized that hulled barley-enriched whole grain lowers down hypercholesterolemia, further improving cholesterol levels by regulating bile acid production leading to its storage in peripheral tissues and lowers down the expression of HMG-COA reductase, which leads to increase in the liver expression of AMP-kinase alpha, low-density lipoprotein receptors, liver X receptor, and peroxisome proliferator-activated receptor alpha [25].

9. Conclusion

Barley (*Hordeum vulgare* L.) is the world's fourth most significant cereal grain, with the greatest fiber composition, and can be utilized in a variety of industries for a variety of uses. Depending on phytonutrients such as glucan, phenolics, flavonoid, lignans, tocols, sitosterol, and folic, regular consumption of whole wheat grain and its hydroethanolic extracts decrease the risk of chronic ailments (hyperglycemia, malignancy, overweight, cardiac disease, and so on). Barley and its products in recent years have gained an importance due to its counteractive components, which play potent role against cardiovascular diseases by lowering down the oxidative stress and improving high-density lipoprotein, further lowering down low-density lipoprotein, VLDL ratios, further regulating insulin levels and lowering down the spike in blood glucose levels, showing potent antioxidative and cardiovascular functions.

Author details

Madiha Khan Niazi[1*], Zainab Saeed[1], Sahar Imran[1] and Farooq Hassan[2]

1 University Institute of Diet and Nutritional Sciences, Faculty of Allied Health Sciences, The University of Lahore, Pakistan

2 Tibb PHC (Punjab Healthcare Commission), Lahore, Pakistan

*Address all correspondence to: dr.madihaniazi@gmail.com

References

[1] Guglielmo M, Lin A, Dey D, Baggiano A, Fusini L, Muscogiuri G, et al. Epicardial fat and coronary artery disease: Role of cardiac imaging. Atherosclerosis. 2021;**321**:30-38

[2] Csige I, Ujvárosy D, Szabó Z, Lőrincz I, Paragh G, Harangi M, et al. The impact of obesity on the cardiovascular system. Journal of Diabetes Research. 2018;**546**:1-12

[3] Tang J, Zheng JS, Fang L, Jin Y, Cai W, Li D. Tea consumption and mortality of all cancers, CVD and all causes: A meta-analysis of eighteen prospective cohort studies. British Journal of Nutrition. 2015;**114**(5):673-683

[4] Hejazi E, Emamat H, Sharafkhah M, Saidpour A, Poustchi H, Sepanlou S, et al. Dietary acid load and mortality from all causes, CVD and cancer: Results from the Golestan cohort study. British Journal of Nutrition. 2022;**128**(2):237-243

[5] Nangia R, Singh H, Kaur K. Prevalence of cardiovascular disease (CVD) risk factors. Medical Journal Armed Forces India. 2016;**72**(4):315-319

[6] Balali-Mood M, Naseri K, Tahergorabi Z, Khazdair MR, Sadeghi M. Toxic mechanisms of five heavy metals: Mercury, lead, chromium, cadmium, and arsenic. Frontiers in Pharmacology. 2021;**12**:643972

[7] Onishi K. Total management of chronic obstructive pulmonary disease (COPD) as an independent risk factor for cardiovascular disease. Journal of Cardiology. 2017;**70**(2):128-134

[8] Cosselman KE, Navas-Acien A, Kaufman JD. Environmental factors in cardiovascular disease. Nature Reviews. Cardiology. 2015;**12**(11):627-642

[9] Sidhu GS, Ward C, Ferdinand KC. Racial disparity in atherosclerotic cardiovascular disease in hospitalized patients with diabetes 2005-2015: Potential warning signs for future US public health. American Journal of Preventive Cardiology. 2020;**4**:100095

[10] Keteepe-Arachi T, Sharma S. Cardiovascular disease in women: Understanding symptoms and risk factors. European Cardiology Review. 2017;**12**(1):10

[11] Zubair F, Nawaz SK, Nawaz A, Nangyal H, Amjad N, Khan MS. Prevalence of cardiovascular diseases in Punjab, Pakistan: A cross-sectional study. Journal of Public Health. 2018;**26**(5):523-529

[12] Einarson TR, Acs A, Ludwig C, Panton UH. Prevalence of cardiovascular disease in type 2 diabetes: A systematic literature review of scientific evidence from across the world in 2007-2017. Cardiovascular Diabetology. 2018;**17**(1):1-9

[13] Chauhan S, Aeri BT. The rising incidence of cardiovascular diseases in India: Assessing its economic impact. European Journal of Preventive Cardiology. 2015;**4**(4):735-740

[14] Woldemichael MD. Importance, biology, epidemiology, and management of loose smut (Ustilago nuda) of barley (*Hordeum vulgare*): A review. East African Journal of Sciences. 2019;**13**(1):89-108

[15] Wang Y, Ren X, Sun D, Sun G. Origin of worldwide cultivated barley

revealed by NAM-1 gene and grain protein content. Frontiers in Plant Science. 2015;**6**(3):1-12. DOI: 10.3389/fpls.2015.00803

[16] Kumar D, Narwal S, Kharub AS, Singh GP. Scope of food barley research and development in India. Wheat and Barley Research. 2018;**10**(3):166-172. Available from: http://epubs.icar.org.in/ejournal/index.php/JWR

[17] Naeem M, Farooq S, Hussain M. The impact of different weed management systems on weed flora and dry biomass production of barley grown under various barley-based cropping systems. Plants. 2022;**11**(6):718

[18] Zeng Y, Pu X, Yang J, et al. Preventive and therapeutic role of functional ingredients of barley grass for chronic diseases in human beings. Oxidative Medicine and Cellular Longevity. 2018;**7**(1):1-15. DOI: 10.1155/2018/3232080.3232080

[19] Kuczyńska A, Cardenia V, Ogrodowicz P, Kempa M, Rodriguez-Estrada MT, Mikołajczak K. Effects of multiple abiotic stresses on lipids and sterols profile in barley leaves (*Hordeum vulgare L.*). Plant Physiology and Biochemistry. 2019;**141**(23):215-224. DOI: 10.1016/j.plaphy.2019.05.033

[20] Jin Y, Li P, Wang F. β-Glucans as potential immunoadjuvants: A review on the adjuvanticity, structure-activity relationship and receptor recognition properties. Vaccine. 2018;**36**(35):5235-5244. DOI: 10.1016/j.vaccine.2018.07.038

[21] Idehen E, Tang Y, Sang S. Bioactive phytochemicals in barley. Journal of Food and Drug Analysis. 2017;**25**(1):148-161. DOI: 10.1016/j.jfda.2016.08.002

[22] Sawicki CM, McKay DL, McKeown NM, Dallal G, Chen CY, Blumberg JB. Phytochemical pharmacokinetics and bioactivity of oat and barley flour: A randomized crossover trial. Nutrients. 2016;**8**(12):813. DOI: 10.3390/nu8120813

[23] Martínez M, Motilva MJ, de Las Hazas MC, Romero MP, Vaculova K, Ludwig IA. Phytochemical composition and β-glucan content of barley genotypes from two different geographic origins for human health food production. Food Chemistry. 2018;**245**(117):61-70. DOI: 10.1016/j.foodchem.2017.09.026

[24] Özcan MM, Aljuhaimi F, Uslu N. Effect of malt process steps on bioactive properties and fatty acid composition of barley, green malt and malt grains. Journal of Food Science and Technology. 2018;**55**(1):226-232. DOI: 10.1007/s13197-017-2920-1

[25] Zhang H, Zhang N, Xiong Z, Wang G, Xia Y, Lai P, et al. Structural characterization and rheological properties of β-D-glucan from hull-less barley (*Hordeum vulgare* L. var. nudum Hook. f.). Phytochemistry. 2018;**155**(67):155-163. DOI: 10.1016/j.phytochem.2018.08.004

[26] Sima P, Vannucci L, Vetvicka V. β-Glucans and cholesterol. International Journal of Molecular Medicine. 2018;**41**(4):1799-1808. DOI: 10.3892/ijmm.2018.3411

[27] Jabeur I, Martins N, Barros L, Calhelha RC, Vaz J, Achour L, et al. Contribution of the phenolic composition to the antioxidant, anti-inflammatory and antitumor potential of Equisetum giganteum L. and Tilia platyphyllos Scop. Food & Function. 2017;**8**(3):975-984. Available from: https://pubs.rsc.org/en/content/articlelanding/2017/fo/c6fo01778a

[28] Hutchinson SA, Lianto P, Moore JB, Hughes TA, Thorne JL. Phytosterols

inhibit side-chain oxysterol mediated activation of LXR in breast cancer cells. International Journal of Molecular Sciences. 2019;**20**(13):3241-3254. DOI: 10.3390/ijms20133241

[29] Şahin Y, Karakas FP. Chemical composition of einkorn (ssp.), emmer (), and spelt (). In: Ancient Wheats 2022. Springer. pp. 119-145, Cham

[30] Punia S, Siroha AK, Sandhu KS, Kaur M. Rheological behavior of wheat starch and barley resistant starch (type IV) blends and their starch noodles making potential. International Journal of Biological Macromolecules. 2019;**130**(34):595-604. DOI: 10.1016/j.ijbiomac.2019.03.009

[31] Zhang J, Xiao X, Dong Y, Shi L, Xu T, Wu F. The anti-obesity effect of fermented barley extracts with lactobacillus plantarum dy-1 and Saccharomyces cerevisiae in diet induced obese rats. Food & Function. 2017;**8**(3):1132-1143. Available from: https://pubs.rsc.org/en/content/articlelanding/2017/fo/c6fo01350c

[32] Guo H, Lin S, Lu M, Gong JD, Wang LU, Zhang Q, et al. Characterization, in vitro binding properties, and inhibitory activity on pancreatic lipase of β-glucans from different Qingke (Tibetan hulless barley) cultivars. International Journal of Biological Macromolecules. 2018;**120**(33):2517-2522. DOI: 10.1016/j.ijbiomac.2018.09.023

[33] Fritsche S, Wang X, Jung C. Recent advances in our understanding of tocopherol biosynthesis in plants: An overview of key genes, functions, and breeding of vitamin E improved crops. Antioxidants. 2017;**6**(4):99-121. Available from: https://www.mdpi.com/2076-3921/6/4/99

[34] Liao Z, Cai H, Xu Z, Wang J, Qiu C, Xie J, et al. Protective role of antioxidant huskless barley extracts on TNF-α-induced endothelial dysfunction in human vascular endothelial cells. Oxidative Medicine and Cellular Longevity. 2018;**15**(2):1-12. DOI: 10.1155/2018/3846029

[35] Gangopadhyay N, Rai DK, Brunton NP, Gallagher E, Hossain MB. Antioxidant-guided isolation and mass spectrometric identification of the major polyphenols in barley (*Hordeum vulgare*) grain. Food Chemistry. 2016;**210**(33):212-220

[36] Ma Y, Wang P, Wang M, Sun M, Gu Z, Yang R. GABA mediates phenolic compounds accumulation and the antioxidant system enhancement in germinated hulless barley under NaCl stress. Food Chemistry. 2019;**270**(39):593-601. DOI: 10.1021/jf802846x

[37] Zhu F. Anthocyanins in cereals: Composition and health effects. Food Research International. 2018;**109**(31):232-249. DOI: 10.1016/j.foodres.2018.04.015

[38] Casieri V, Matteucci M, Cavallini C, Torti M, Torelli M, Lionetti V. Long-term intake of pasta containing barley (1-3) beta-D-glucan increases neovascularization-mediated cardioprotection through endothelial upregulation of vascular endothelial growth factor and parkin. Scientific Reports. 2017;**7**(1):1-6. DOI: 10.1038/s41598-017-13949-1

[39] Tong LT, Zhong K, Liu L, Zhou X, Qiu J, Zhou S. Effects of dietary hull-less barley β-glucan on the cholesterol metabolism of hypercholesterolemic hamsters. Food Chemistry. 2015;**169**(23):344-349. DOI: 10.1016/j.foodchem.2014.07.157

[40] Crowley T, Fitzpatrick JM, Kuijper T, Cryan JF, O'Toole O, O'Leary OF, et al. Modulation of TLR3/TLR4 inflammatory signaling by the GABAB receptor agonist baclofen in glia and immune cells: Relevance to therapeutic effects in multiple sclerosis. Frontiers in Cellular Neuroscience. 2015;**9**(2):284-293. Available from: https://www.ncbi.nlm.nih.gov/pmc/articles/PMC4516894/

[41] Middleton EA, Weyrich AS, Zimmerman GA. Platelets in pulmonary immune responses and inflammatory lung diseases. Physiological Reviews. 2016;**96**(4):1211-1259. DOI: 10.1152/physrev.00038.2015

[42] Health Canada. Eating Well with Canada's Food Guide. 2007. Available from: http://www.hc-sc.gc.ca/fn-an/foodguide-aliment/order-commander/index-eng.php. [Accessed: January 16, 2014]

[43] Barone Gibbs B, Hivert MF, Jerome GJ, Kraus WE, Rosenkranz SK, Schorr EN, et al. Physical activity as a critical component of first-line treatment for elevated blood pressure or cholesterol: Who, what, and how?: A scientific statement from the American Heart Association. Hypertension. 2021;**78**(2):e26-e37

[44] Bacchetti T, Tullii D, Masciangelo S, Gesuita R, Skrami E, Brugè F, et al. Effect of a barley-vegetable soup on plasma carotenoids and biomarkers of cardiovascular disease. Journal of Clinical Biochemistry and Nutrition. 2015;**57**(1):66-73. DOI: 10.3164/jcbn.15-11